The
POWER
of
LETTERS

A COMPILATION OF LETTERS SHOWING WHAT
A POSITIVE MINDSET CAN ACHIEVE

By Team Inspire

Disclaimer

A catalogue of this book is available in the British Library.

JUST IMAGINE...

...how a few simple words could change your entire day

We wanted to share a few things we have learnt over the years and hope they may help you focus on what's important when you think things aren't going your way. Take it from us, we have been there, and we are sharing our tales with you today.

Don't worry so much, as it will always turn out just fine. Even when it doesn't exactly, you will always find a way to get through it. So just enjoy the journey and have faith.

Embrace every opportunity, don't let fear of failure hold you back. You're never too old to start something new today. What's the worst that could happen? You won't know until you try.

And finally, for now...don't wait to be asked ...sometimes you have to give yourself permission to just give things a go. Have fun, you will definitely surprise yourself.

We have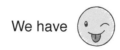

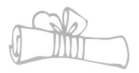

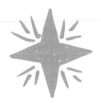

DEDICATION

The challenge was set. A small team from Pitney Bowes, a global shipping and mailing company, entered The Prince's Trust Million Makers 2021 to raise funds to build better futures for the next generation and support young adults back to work through training and education.

This small group of people volunteered much of their personal time to become Team Inspire. This team demonstrated the power of coming together with heart, humanity, and focus. Taking a blank sheet of paper, we began with our collective imaginations and soon created the concept for this book to raise valuable funds for this noteworthy charity.

At the time of entering the challenge, our company, Pitney Bowes, was 101 years old. Having witnessed changes in technology, in how we work and in the way we support learning for all, we decided to link our idea to who we have been, and who we are now. Our book *The Power of Letters* is our way to rejuvenate the written word, remind us of the power of what's ahead, and stay thankful for the support we received both from The Prince's Trust and Pitney Bowes for this unique opportunity.

Our book, *The Power of Letters*, is dedicated to all who have ever had a challenging moment, who may have not always felt they could, but they did. Who knew that if they gave it their best – no matter what – with help and support, they realised that they could achieve so much. Through adversity, big or small, no matter what that looks like, anything is possible with a positive mindset.

These pages may make a difference to you or to others you may wish to inspire.

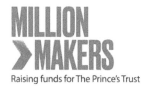

MILLION >MAKERS

Raising funds for The Prince's Trust

What you hold in your hand is a collection of letters, showcasing the value of what a POSITIVE MINDSET CAN ACHIEVE

INTRODUCTION

The Prince's Trust believes that every young person should have the chance to succeed, no matter what their background or the challenges they are facing. They help those from disadvantaged communities and those facing the greatest adversity by supporting them to build the confidence and skills to live, learn and earn.

The courses offered by The Trust help young people aged 11-30 to develop essential life skills, get ready for work and access job opportunities. They support them to find work because having a job or running a business can lead to a more stable and fulfilling life.

Since The Trust was founded by The Prince of Wales in 1976, they have helped more than a million young people across the UK.

And now, we at Team Inspire want to do our part, too. With The Power of Letters, we want to raise funds for The Prince's Trust, because young adults deserve a better future with our help through education and training to help them into jobs.

What you hold in your hand is a collection of letters and poems, showcasing the value of what a positive mindset can achieve. To help remind people to believe in themselves. With a positive frame of mind, you can achieve anything you want. This book shares real-life experiences from everyday people (some famous) young and old for a diversity of thought across different life journeys.

Challenges can come in all shapes and sizes, and mental health in all its guises does not discriminate. It can happen to anyone, any race, gender and at any age, with varying impact. No matter what you are going through and dealing with, it is always good to know that you are not alone. Our collection of letters will inspire you and remind you that others have triumphed over adversity, and you will, too.

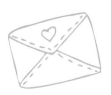

HOW TO GET THE BEST OUT OF THIS BOOK

There is no right or wrong way to read this book: you can read cover to cover, or you can flip to a random page for inspiration. You can read on a train, on a plane, at home under a pile of blankets, in the bath (just don't drop it!), sat in a waiting room or on a beach. You can call a friend and read a bit to them, or you can buy them their own copy and read together. However you choose to read, let this book become a friend to inspire and comfort you when you need it.

We believe by learning from other people's experiences and reflections, you can find hope.

Even from adversity and by maintaining a positive mindset, you can achieve an optimistic future.

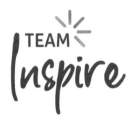

TRIGGER WARNING

Please know that to help us create this book we asked for letter contributions to gain real peoples' experiences. Our request was for stories that would help many from the ages of 16+.

Many of the letters or poems are about important topics that for some may be uncomfortable to read or today may cause offense. They cover topics that many people suffer in silence. We always wanted to share real life experiences. In each letter or poem, we saw that with strength and focus coupled with a positive mindset you can achieve anything, especially in times of anxiety or darkness.

Some subjects shared by our contributors do range from different forms of mental health issues, physical and mental abuse, and various feelings and levels of despair.

At the end of this book, we provide contact numbers of organisations that offer helpline support for a variety of issues found in this book.

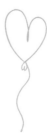

CONTENTS

These quotes popped out to us. Jump ahead and read the letter or poem in full. What catches your eye? What words speak to you?

"Keep going. No matter how hard it may seem. Even if you feel it's the end of the world. It is not the end." 50

"We only get one life, so let's both make it an amazing one. Create the life you want to live. What's stopping you?" 52

"If you want something badly enough, just keep plugging away and you'll get there in the end." 55

"It takes courage to ask for help and even greater courage to accept it. It is not a weakness but a strength." 57

"Do not see the pain and struggle as something to avoid or fear – no, it is quite the opposite. On the other side lies your greatest and most powerful self." 59

"Believe and achieve." 60

"Dreams aren't just for sleeping. They are sneak peeks of what is yet to come." 64

"No matter what was in my path, I wanted to live life on my own terms." 66

"We need others to make a stand to evoke change." 71

"It's ok to take some time out. Until you feel yourself once more." 74

"Look within yourself. Know that your dreams and hopes are valid and that only you can make them come true." 75

"Adversity has taught me that the potential to feel better and do better is always there – it is up to us to align to it and to chase it." 78

"Every application and interview really is a learning experience." 80

"Stand on your beach and throw that starfish back in." 83

"Try to find that little bit of light, the good. It's there somewhere, I promise. Grab onto it. Let it carry you through the darkness, because you'll come out on the other side soon." 87

"Because, you can do anything. You're you. A youey you, blowing your bubbles – up, up, up. And nobody else can blow bubbles like you." 91

Optimistic Futures

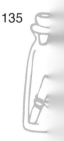

Reflections

HOPES
and
DREAMS

TO ANYONE UNDERESTIMATING THE VALUE OF KINDNESS –

It's 1995, and every weekend I catch the bus into Bolton town center. I meet with my cousin and a few other black friends. We usually spend the afternoon in The Water Place, a swimming center with slides, a wave machine, and numerous pools.

I'd just got my first pair of "cool" trainers, white and gold Adidas Galaxy. I'm sure my parents had got them from the Littlewoods catalogue and probably were paying over a period of time.

There were various groups that used to hang out in the town center, and most of them were older teenagers from different parts of Bolton. One Saturday, I had to leave early, so I went to get showered and changed on my own. I'm in the changing rooms getting dressed, and that's when I hear it

"It's that black twat with the trainers."

Next thing I know, I've taken a beating, lip bust, one lens fallen out of my glasses and my new trainers stolen. It all happened in a flash, and I stood little chance against a group.

Cue me walking to the bus station feeling very sorry for myself in just my socks. I probably walked past 30 people until I was stopped by a woman. She looked at me, didn't say a word, other than follow me. Reflecting back, following strangers isn't the most streetwise, but it turned out to be a sensible choice.

She took me to Shoe Zone and bought me a £12 pair of basic white trainers and a pack of socks. I asked her name; she was called Helen. "Why did you help?" She said:

"Sometimes, you have to trust your gut. You don't look like a bad kid, but you're in a bad situation. It's easy to ignore those in need, but kindness doesn't cost much and can make a big difference. You won't have wet feet and your parents worried when you get home."

The trainers were the least cool pair you've ever seen, but I walked to the bus station like they were coated in gold. Once on the bus, I started to worry about how to tell my parents. They probably knew, but I made up some excuses, and I saved up my pocket money and bought a cheaper similar looking version from the shop that would become Streetwise Sports a few years later.

Why share a story from 25 years ago?

Well, I can't put a price on Helen's kindness. I've never met her since to say thank you. But her faith in me is something that I've kept close to my heart through my journey.

I might have been a victim of racism, violence and theft on that day, but in the adversity, I found hope and optimism in one single moment of kindness.

Never underestimate what kindness can do for someone in a moment of need.

Lee Chambers,

Psychologist and Wellbeing Consultant at Essentialise

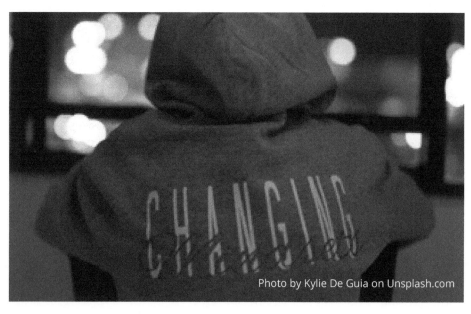

Photo by Kylie De Guia on Unsplash.com

TO ANYONE DOUBTING THEMSELVES –

If only…

If only I had the courage to ask him out.
If only I had done that before.
If only I had not said those words out loud.
If only I could take back what I did, I didn't mean it.
If only I got up earlier. Went to bed on time.
If only I said more of what I loved about them.
If only I didn't hurt myself.
If only the scars would heal quicker.
If only people would see me.
If only people didn't see me, and I could be invisible.
If only I was stronger.
If only I was able to cry and tell someone.
If only I knew what it was to be young. When I was.
If only I was older, I'd be taken more seriously.
If only I would stop wasting my time with – if only.

When you add up the times you think like this, a lifetime can pass you by, then in a moment, you are saying … "If only I had."

Don't let these two words stop you from finding out what you can be at any stage in your life. Just know you can be. Anyone can.

I wish I could see you achieve all that you can be, if only

With love,

Hina Sharma

> **Our minds are powerful. As quickly as we can be beaten down, we CAN recover.** BRIGHTER DAYS ARE AHEAD.

TO ANYONE IN A DARK PLACE RIGHT NOW –

My name is Lee. I am 38 years old, engaged to my partner of four years and have four beautiful daughters. I have a great job, a lovely family home, the best family you could wish for and a great circle of friends. I am happy.

Six years ago, I didn't think I'd ever write that paragraph.

The thing is most of the things in that paragraph were still true back then. Back in early 2015, I had been married for seven years, had two beautiful daughters, a good job, a great family, including perfect in-laws around me, but things were about to change.

I was married relatively young at 24 and welcomed my first daughter that same year. To my friends, I had it all, and perhaps on paper I did, but inside I was far from happy. For years I lived in denial. When the separation came about, I can't lie and say it was a shock. It hadn't been a happy marriage behind closed doors for several years, and we had been clinging on to nothing for the sake of our children for far too long. My wife was a good person; she gave me the two greatest things in my life, and at times I was far from the perfect husband. Here we were, calling time on our marriage with no going back. The decision felt like a weight lifted off my shoulders. I could get through this, surely.

One day I went to work knowing that when I came home, my wife and children would be gone. Nothing, and I mean nothing, could prepare me for what came next. For seven years, I had put my key in the door to the sound of little footsteps running towards me, screams of "Daddy," followed by a massive hug. This time, the footsteps didn't come. There was nothing but silence. I walked into my empty house and past their bedroom. Their bunk beds were perfectly made with their teddies set out as they always were.

Everything hit me there and then, the magnitude of what was happening. Guilt, fear and sadness overcame me, and I had never felt more alone. That night, there was no bedtime story, only a Facetime call seeing my girls in another house. To them, it was an exciting new adventure. To me, it was the most excruciating phone call I'll ever make.

Months went by, and I tried to carry on. The reality was this: days were hard, I struggled to focus at work, and my productivity duly suffered. I was able to bullsh*t my way through a lot of stuff, but I was dropping plates, my mind preoccupied with how I was going to get myself through this mess.

Nights were when I struggled the most. Loneliness is the worst emotion I've ever felt, and I felt it deeply during those nights at home, surrounded by photos of my girls. Turning the TV off and walking past their bedroom to get to mine was the hardest ten-meter walk you can imagine, repeated each night. The silence was the worst, nobody to talk to, no laughter, no cries, no splashing in the bath, nothing. I lived for the three nights a week they stayed with me.

Months rolled by, and I slumped deeper into depression. I lost friends along the way; I was horrible to be around looking back. My dad, not famed for his sensitive side, took me to Spain for a few days to watch a football match. He sat opposite me with a beer saying, "It'll all be okay, you know." "Shut up, Dad, I don't need counselling. I'm fine." Of course, I wasn't, but that's not the manly thing to admit, is it?

Something had to change.

The biggest mistake I made was trying to get through it all alone. One big fake front was all it was, and that's mentally exhausting. You can't keep that up, trust me. The feeling I got when I sought counselling was liberating. I got it all out. I wanted to get better and break this cycle.

One piece of advice I'd give anyone going through something similar is don't try to convince yourself that every negative situation has a positive element. Accept the fact that sometimes life can just be bloody hard, and it can hit you from different angles all at once. No matter how strong you think you are, anyone can suffer, and nobody is immune. If you need to cry, cry. Crying is massively therapeutic. We are human beings, and emotions are perfectly normal. If you have a good family, lean on them. If you have a best friend, talk to them.

Our minds are powerful. As quickly as we can be beaten down, we CAN recover. Brighter days are ahead. You've just got to hang on to that thought.

You can't do it alone, but it starts with a decision only you can make.

I am aware that as a man, this can be especially hard. We have thousands of years of evolution telling us to be strong, man up, pull ourselves together.

Break-ups are hard; adjusting to a new routine with our children is arguably harder. It was for me. What I want you to know is that others have been through it, are going through it and will understand that you are going through it.

As Rocky Balboa once said, "***The world ain't all sunshine and rainbows. It's a very mean and nasty place, and I don't care how tough you are; it will beat you to your knees and keep you there permanently if you let it. You, me or nobody is gonna hit as hard as life. But it ain't about how hard you hit, it's about how hard you can get hit and keep moving forward. How much you can take and keep moving forward. That's how winning is done.***"

I have that quote framed above my desk at home, and I read it each day to remind myself of where I have been and where I want to go.

There was a point I almost gave up, but then I thought of my children and remembered who was watching.

I hope this helped in some way, and even though I don't know you, these words provide some hope.

Look after yourself.

Lee

To My Fellow Dreamers –

First of all, I hope you are fine and healthy. I would like to share my personal journey with you about my hopes and dreams.

When the pandemic started, I was studying for my college entry exams, and I lost all of the motivation. I knew I had to force myself to study, but I just couldn't. Nothing seemed to be helping. Day after day, I was getting more worried that I'd fail in all subjects, so I tried my best to get up and said, "Listen, if you want to get into that college you always dreamed of, you have to study." I started studying a bit until my exams arrived. I did my exams – yes, I was nervous, and yes, I had that anxiety that I would not pass. But I believed myself that I would pass, and if I didn't, well, I would still be proud because at least I tried to study especially during the pandemic.

The day arrived when I received my marks, and out of ten subjects, I passed eight. I had to redo two of them to get into the college I always dreamed of. I already did three of them, and tomorrow I will do the fourth and last exam. I had hope, I still have hope, and I will keep hoping that I will get into that college. Why stop chasing a dream that I have been chasing my whole life? That is why I keep on doing what I can to get into this college.

You should do the same, from my experience I hope you took something with you that can help you chase your goals, keep having hope, keep chasing your dreams until it becomes a reality and anything you really wish.

I wish you all the success for your future.

Yours truly,

Sefora Bonello

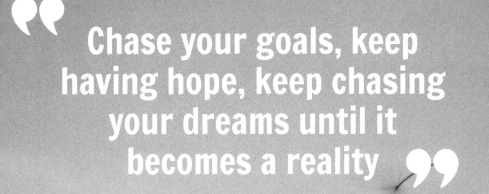

Chase your goals, keep having hope, keep chasing your dreams until it becomes a reality

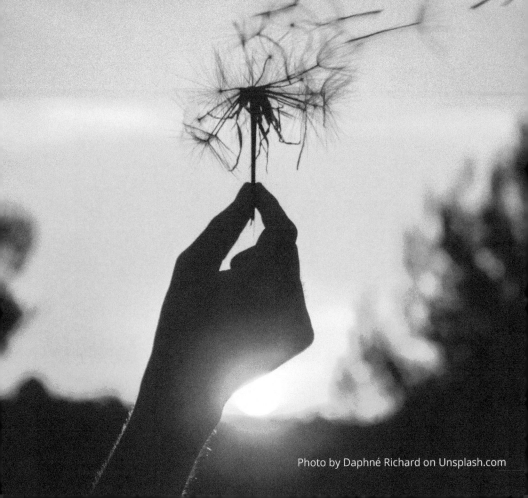

TO ANYONE STRUGGLING –

... I know how the dark place feels
I've felt it's cold; Know the bitter of its heat.
That wanting to retreat.
Back against the wall with nowhere to flee,
To be free
From the dark surround.
The sound
Of nothing when you're in a crowd.
Then the suddenness of any noise;
Any noise is way too loud.
The choke of tongue twisting conversation
In relation
to trauma that cuts deep.
I taste the sweat, seep
From my pores.
The trauma is mine… not yours
So y'all know not what your sniggering Is triggering.
Then, you're wondering why you don't see or hear me for weeks.
My texting speaks
More than my mouth in that time.
The sublime
Sound of painful solace easing me into comfort to engage with the world
yet again…

But, here's the thing…

I also know the joy that makes a feral cry sing
A melody with textures so dope
It conjures up the brightness of tangible hope.
Keeping me from the rope

Allowing the mechanisms to cope
In ways I hadn't the tools to access Before.
Before, existence
Now, life.
I live.
Now, is gifted.
Before…

…

Before, life was a task.
A massive ask.
A chore.
I wore
A mask of many me's.
And there were many a me at one time.
Now there's no need.
There's a rhythm and a rhyme
In my every step.
Every step
A step closer to another place I know.
A place of light.
I glow.
No cold.
No fight.
Where the heat tastes fresh and the retreat is healthy.
Where emotions aren't rich, they're wealthy.
I bathe in the sound of a peaceful noise from my inner voice
That chokes with laughter as I speak of my past woes.
And so the story goes, I can speak of them now as I do, without shame.
Without cursing my name
Or the constant self-blame.
All this, I overcame…
… And so can you.

Nicholas Pinnock,
actor, producer, mental health advocate and activist

To ANYONE WHO FEELS LIKE GIVING UP –

This is my story of how I became a Mum. It was a long journey, and like most things worth fighting for, it was a hard one. It took us six years, several failed IVF cycles, three miscarriages and a selfless surrogate to bring our beautiful son, Spencer John Wilson, into the world.

> My path to motherhood was full of heartbreak and pain. But it was also full of hope and perseverance as I knew it would all be worth it in the end.

Soon after my husband Ryan and I married, we decided to try for a family. Being in our early thirties then, we naively thought it would be easy. But after about a year, we knew something wasn't right. And so, we started IVF.

It was a roller coaster of emotions. Some weeks I felt despair, anger, and guilt. Other weeks, I was optimistic and full of adrenalin. Working through those contrasting emotions for years was often exhausting.

After several failed and cancelled IVF cycles and a miscarriage, we changed to an implantation specialist who diagnosed me with having a thin endometrium lining. As the wallpaper of the uterus, the lining is crucial to becoming pregnant and sustaining a pregnancy.

At our appointment, he hit us with the hard truth: thin linings are rare, usually genetic, and difficult to fix. He then told us surrogacy was our best chance of having a baby. But not ready to close the door on being pregnant myself, we pushed ahead with a transfer on a thin lining and became pregnant. The high was enormous.

At our first scan at 7.5 weeks, we had the devastating news our baby's heartbeat was too slow. Two days later, at our follow-up scan, she had passed. We were absolutely crushed. Shortly after a D&C procedure, our specialist called with the biopsy results. The baby had been genetically normal. The baby was a girl. I wish I hadn't found out the gender. It made the loss more real and more heartbreaking.

The overriding takeaway, though, was that this loss confirmed that the issue was me. It was really hard to accept. But with the support of my family and friends and a wonderful counsellor, I was able to work through the grief of never being able to carry my own baby and to accept our next chapter – surrogacy.

With surrogacy a difficult process in Australia, we started in Canada with Julie, a selfless woman who felt compelled to help us. It was a long flight (18 hours) for the transfer, but it was such an important milestone.

What happened next still haunts me. The day of the transfer, our specialist told us the devastating news that the container of embryos we had transported was empty. With a pounding heart and almost breathless, I kept asking him, "What do you mean by empty? Who can we call?"

He looked at me sadly, spoke to me in a gentle voice. There was no one to call. The embryos were gone. We knew that there was a standard protocol for transporting embryos, so what happened to us was extremely rare. Our lawyers and fertility clinics in Melbourne and Toronto had never heard of this ever happening.

This was one of the lowest points during our journey.

It was at this time I saw a psychologist who used hypnotherapy and cognitive behavioral therapy (CBT). She recommended that instead of fixating on what I didn't have, to focus on what I did. And to try, as hard as it was, to not let the infertility consume me. Yes, it was a significant part of my life, but I shouldn't let it be my identity. I shouldn't let it have that power over me. There is no question that adopting the CBT techniques helped to reshape my mindset and build my resilience.

We pursued surrogacy next in the United States, our last hurrah. We had an instant bond with our beautiful US surrogate, Leigha, and her husband, Josh. I will always be in awe of surrogates. How someone who doesn't know you hears your story and feels compelled to help you.

Our first transfer failed, but our second transfer worked. We heard the heartbeat at our 8-week scan, and we all felt at peace. But at our 10-week scan, we learned the heartbreaking news our baby had passed.

At this point, I resigned myself to thinking we would never have a child. I wanted to scream and cry and be done with the whole thing. With every setback, I had faith. But this time, the fight had vanished. I was struggling to move past the fact we were here again.

But we had some good embryos left, and our surrogate Leigha was determined to keep going. Ryan encouraged me, repeating everything the doctor had said about how the miscarriage was rare (subchorionic hematoma) and unlikely to happen again. We decided to try one last time.

Leigha felt anxious, but she charged into the final transfer giving it her all. It reminded me of a quote from Atticus Finch from one of my favorite books, To Kill a Mockingbird*: "*Real courage is when you know you're licked before you begin, but you begin anyway and see it through no matter what.*"

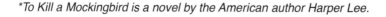

Nine months later, our beautiful son
Spencer was born.

Michael Jordan once famously said his late father taught him to always "take a negative and turn it into a positive." I think MJ is onto something.

And the greatest positive? Spencer, of course. And the immense gratitude and love we have for him. For the first six months of his life, not a day went by when I didn't cry every morning when I picked him up out of his cot. Overwhelmed with emotion, the tears always fell. The poor kid probably didn't know what to think as I saturated him with my salty tears. But I couldn't believe that he was actually here. That we had finally been blessed with a child. Our own little miracle.

Kirsten McLennan

*To Kill a Mockingbird is a novel by the American author Harper Lee.

" Real courage is when you know you're licked before you begin but you begin anyway... "

To ANYONE FEELING BURDENED BY EXPECTATIONS,

As I sit here writing my letter, I realize that I grow more anxious and self-critical by the second. "No. That's too wordy," or "No; too bland!" Further and further, I continue to berate myself until I buckle under the weight of my own expectation. If you take nothing else from this letter but the fact that it is okay to fail, it is okay to be afraid, then I think I have done my part.

Growing up, I was told all too often that I was brimming with potential or that I was incredibly talented. Yet I dreaded every single one of my report cards and PTAs.

If I had so much potential, why was I failing in so many classes? Why was I drawn into books and video games instead of focusing on my studies?

Looking back, I realize now that I actually dreaded studying. If I put in the effort and failed, then I really wasn't as 'special' as everyone said I was. It was easier to act as if I didn't care than to admit that I was just scared.

My parents loved me then as they love me now, and they only ever tried their best to make sure that I had a good future. They believed that talking to me and saying that I was talented but lazy would inspire me to try better. Spoiler alert: it didn't.

Their words manifested a pernicious life of its own and turned it into one of the many voices of doubt which plagued me. It told me that I would fail, that I wasn't good enough, that I was doing it all wrong. It never felt enough, and I knew it wasn't my mother's or father's intention, but the doubt and pressure bubbled inside me until I felt directionless.

When I decided to change, it was because of the kind of person I wanted to be, and not because of anything that someone else said. I continued writing fiction because I was good at it, no matter how skeptical or doubtful my parents were. As more and more people began to enjoy my work, I gained the confidence that I so desperately needed to struggle on.

It was at the end of October in 2020, after my debut novel was out, when my parents said the words I never knew I wanted to hear: "I am no longer worried about you."

Yet still, expectation and doubt are something I struggle with, and they will continue to accompany me. Expectation from my readers, my parents, my friends, and worst of all: myself.

So, I learnt two important things: it was okay to fail, it was okay to make a mistake. I still had all the tools necessary to stand up and try again. It was okay to be afraid of failing, but that didn't mean I shouldn't at least try.

Expectation is the culmination of all things which tell us how high we can rise, but it isn't often addressed how far we will fall if we fail. The higher the climb, the more treacherous the fall may seem. So, cushion that lending with supportive friends and remove the jagged voices that say, "I told you so." Find family that encourages and supports you because they will be the proverbial arms that catch you when you fall.

Expectation can be so debilitating and scary because of potential failure, so learn to accept failure as part of it. In fact, I would not have made it where I am without failing all the time.

At the age of 19, I was diagnosed with Generalized Anxiety Disorder. It is not something that can be cured, but I have learnt to live with it. If the voices whisper portent words that I will fail, I will remind them that it is okay.

I will not tell any of you that mental illness is something that can be easily overcome with an anecdotal letter from some random guy. This isn't that kind of letter. My point is that no one's life is set in stone and that it is always possible to find something that makes you live up to all that expectation if you just embrace the fall.

Kian N. Ardalan

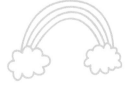

**Because it's only in falling
Do we learn to fly**

TO MY FELLOW ADVENTURERS,

That adventure we call life

We start off by dreaming it
We then learn how to work for it
Then we work for it
Of course, we fall down for it too
And we get up and dust ourselves off for it
We have sleepless nights for it
We have so many challenges for it
We have adventures, new experiences and memories for it
We chase horizons and sunsets for it
What is it ... life
We all have a goal, a dream, and an adventure waiting
We just have to be brave enough
To take the leap into ... the unknown
To be brave enough to chase our horizon
Our moments, our adventures, our achievements and our failures
To believe that when we leap and fall
Our wings will take flight
Because it's only in falling
Do we learn to fly

Emma Ramshaw

DEAR FRIEND,

I hope that as you are reading this, you are in a place of happiness, but if not, that is ok. You are not alone, and you never will be.

Things might be far from perfect, but always remember that you are enough. A few years ago, I was in a very dark and sad place. I went through the scariest and most difficult period of my life.

I was sectioned for over three weeks because of an acute psychotic episode. This was triggered by a break-up, but I was also being hard on myself for not achieving my personal goals at the time, things like owning a property and getting promoted at work became unhealthy obsessions.

I had to take some heavy medication. I continued taking the medication when I got out of the psychiatric ward, and they slowly helped me get better.

Thankfully I am now over the worse of it and am currently living a much happier life.

I am still on medication (quetiapine), but I choose to take this because I know it will prevent me from becoming unwell again. I also attended cognitive behavioral therapy, which helped me so much. Almost every session included tears, but the release was just what I needed, and it made me a better person.

The reason I am telling you these things is because I want you to know that even if you hit rock bottom, you can turn it around. The thing with rock bottom is that you discover the solid, unbreakable, courageous part of yourself that will never be beaten, and you can build on that foundation and make it even better than it once was. You might be hitting the reset button, maybe more than once, but trust me, you will build something to be proud of.

Life can be hard, but life is also very precious. Try and surround yourself with people who make you happy and make you laugh out loud.

I do not regret becoming mentally ill because it took me on a journey that has eventually transformed me into the best version of myself.

Self-care and self-awareness are so important. If you think you need help, always seek it. If you think you can help someone else, be there for them, it might even save their life.

Try not to compare yourselves to others. We are all so beautifully unique as individuals, and your journey is completely different to everyone else's. Embrace your imperfections, your weirdness, your everything.

Try not to be hard on yourself; you are not your thoughts. It might feel like your mind is a storm at times, but this will pass; the sunshine is closer than you think.

You might even be healthier than ever right now, and that's fantastic. Never take your wellbeing for granted, do your best to preserve it. I, unfortunately, had to go through a relapse at one point, caused by a mistake in taking my medication, but also by trying to do too many things that resulted in stress and eventual breakdown.

There are loads of coping mechanisms out there, and I can tell you that some work really well for me. I do plenty of yoga, I try to do meditation when I can, and exercise is often my saving grace. Running, cycling, swimming, and playing football are things that work wonders for my brain. Your best bet is to try as many new things as you can, then you might discover a passion that changes your life.

I hope you have found my little letter helpful, wherever you are.

Thanks for reading, and thanks for being you.

James, 31, from Hertfordshire

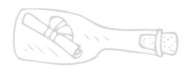

TO ANYONE WHO CAN'T SEE A WAY OUT –

The night he came home drunk is a night I will never forget. His irritation turned to rage and then quickly escalated to violence. As the abuse carried on, I was terrified, knowing my daughter – only a few months old – was sleeping upstairs. I had been frightened of him before, but this night the abuse reached such a horrifying level that I called the police. I'd had enough, and I had my baby girl to think about. He was arrested, and I finally made the decision to leave.

I thought I had escaped the abuse, but I hadn't, and post-separation abuse continued till I had no choice but to stop access and all contact. The police came and went with no convictions despite threats on my life and further violent attacks.

The day I had been dreading finally came, and court proceedings started. As a litigant in person, I was unaware of my rights, and the whole case from start to finish was horrifying. Evidence was ignored, none of the usual procedures were followed, I was spoken down to, and despite my complaints and appeals, I was ignored for months and months. I expected that my daughter and I would be protected by the judiciary system, but instead, our basic rights were breached over and over.

In despair, I reached out to women's charities and others for help.

Soon the realization came that my story wasn't an isolated one, and there were so many others in my position.

I was left furious with a system that was failing the most vulnerable, and that fury I turned into determination and a dream to do something about it. I started by speaking out and telling my story, which has always been a terrifying thing to do as it is illegal to speak out about family law cases. I wanted to campaign to change this amongst other legislation that needed reform.

Soon after, I decided to raise money for a domestic abuse charity, and in order to raise the money, I wanted to climb Ben Nevis. In the following months, others wanted to join me, and we all managed to get a great amount of press coverage for the campaigning and the trek.

Trekking the 1,345m mountain in the rain and cold was worth it as we achieved raising £4,000 for the domestic abuse charity. The personal sense of achievement was greater after everything I had been through and endured. I felt I was standing up for not just myself but so many others who didn't have a voice to be heard. I wanted to make a stand for all those who had suffered abuse and been let down by the system, and I wanted to leave a legacy behind for my daughter that she could be proud of.

Since then, I have taken part in speaking on Times Radio and other podcasts and continue to speak out and campaign for change. My hope is that there will be more law change and that those who need protecting will be protected as they should be. My dream is to see that happen before my daughter is older.

> The only way to make hopes and dreams come true is the determination to make them come true, to persevere even when you are scared, and to never back down when you know something is worth standing for.

Hopes and dreams are what makes change for the better and are what feeds the good in the world we live in.

Charlotte Budd

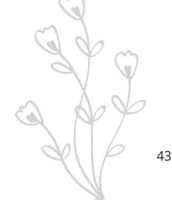

43

I definitely didn't picture this path for myself, BUT I WOULDN'T CHANGE IT FOR THE WORLD.

TO ANYONE TRYING TO FIND THEIR WAY –

There are two things I wish I had been told at the age of 16.

1) You can work for yourself.

You don't need to work *for* someone, and you don't need to approach work in the 'traditional' way. Not anymore. With our current technology, a computer and an internet connection are all you need to earn money. Since the pandemic, even working from home has become the norm. When I started on my career path, working from home was considered lazy: "But you're in your pajamas all day, lying on the sofa – it's not a real job!" Ignore the naysayers. It is a real job. And I wasn't lying on the sofa, or in my pajamas, but that was the attitude of the older generation around me.

2) Achieving a goal that is truly worthwhile is never straightforward.

If goals were straightforward, they wouldn't be considered achievements. There is no easy way to achieve a goal. We often forget that, between the start and the finish line, there'll be missed deadlines, sudden problems that divert your attention; the goal might even change completely. When this happens, don't let yourself feel beaten, unsuccessful, or a failure. It's all about how we respond to these challenges, and if you accept that they are inevitable, you will allow yourself to learn and develop each step of the way. Only those who have the courage to step into unknown territory will achieve their bigger goals in life.

I graduated university aged 22 in 2016 with a 2:1 in Philosophy and English Literature and decided to move to Sheffield with a friend. I had no clue what I wanted to do with myself. I had no job, no money. I was living in a damp-ridden and moldy two-room, downstairs flat, and I had to accept Universal Credit. We had one bed and one sofa – that was our only furniture. This was how I started my journey.

After six months of applying for jobs I didn't actually want, I was humiliated, depressed, and always so tired. I *hated* interviews and their effect on my mental health. I hated having to do work I didn't enjoy. But finances were dwindling.

It was my twin who pushed me onto my journey. He sat me down and asked me what skills I had that I could monetize. At the time, I hardly knew what that meant. I'd always wanted to work with books, but it felt like a pipe dream, something I'd talk about wistfully when walking into a bookshop.

But I did have a skill that I could monetize. I was good at English grammar, and I'd run a student magazine at university. On next to no money, I built a free website and started promoting myself as an editor. I started a business in March 2017 without spending a dime. But I had a lot of learning to do. I knew nothing about running a business, but I was lucky that my older brother did. When I moved back home a few months later, he taught me how to stay on top of my finances and how to file my own taxes. He taught me how to understand all of that confusing business-speak: overheads, sole trader, tax returns, limited company, financial projection, and so on.

It took about a year for the work to come in earnest, but in 2018, I celebrated my first £1k job. That summer, I named my business Softwood Self-Publishing and designed a logo – all of it for free. The plan was to offer every service a writer would need to self-publish their book.

By the end of 2018, at the age of 25, I could afford to move into a three-bed house with my partner and his three sons. Over the next year, I worked harder than ever before, editing manuscripts and scientific papers and writing my own novel at last, despite an arm injury, a half-finished postgraduate course in English Literature, and endless money worries. My anxious brain that had always held me back was starting to unravel and trust that I was on the right path.

Then came the pandemic. The first month was silent. I had no clients and no work booked in, which, by then, was unusual for me. But as the dust settled and we all got used to lockdown, the people began to write. By June 2020, I had so much work that my partner, Nathan, joined the business to run its social media platforms. From there, everything changed. It was no longer just an editing business, with me hidden away at a desk. Nathan helped with admin, emails, promotion, website, and more. He then began to take on his own clients, helping writers promote their books after publication. Before long, my little freelance editing gig became a fully-fledged business with more than one member of staff: we amassed editors, formatters, an amazing cover designer, printers, and a marketer, and I finally self-published my own novel in December 2020.

In 2021, we were running creative writing and self-publishing workshops at book festivals across the UK, and offers of workshops began to come in from overseas, where we were now attracting a large proportion of our clients. We moved to a gorgeous village in Suffolk, got Softwood's first office, and I began to write my second book.

I can summarize the last six years in a few paragraphs, but my path has not been straightforward. I have battled anxiety, financial trouble, serious injury, as well as prejudice against my job. I have run a business while being step-mum to three boys, getting engaged, keeping up with family, and maintaining a household. I can't pretend it's easy – it's exhausting at the best of times. But I've reached my goals a few times now and had to make new ones, and I did this while working for myself. When I was 16, I definitely didn't picture this path for myself, but I wouldn't change it for the world.

Maddy Glenn

Director of Softwood Self-Publishing

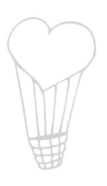

HELLO YOU,

You need to know you are beautiful for who you are. You are the sun from above, shining out of your personality.

You are the best you can be, and everyone loves you for that.

Don't judge or be afraid of who you are or want to be because you are perfect.

Let your ambition and inspirations bring out the best in you.

Carry on doing what you do best, and never forget there is an angel watching over you, protecting you and praising you!

I wanted to let you know how special you are and remind you that you are a very important part of our wonderful world.

So go ahead, imagine what you want to achieve, feel it, see it in your mind.

Remember it like something that has already happened.

Feel how you will feel when you have already achieved it, and it will come into being.

That's how the magic happens.

Sam Livermore

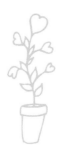

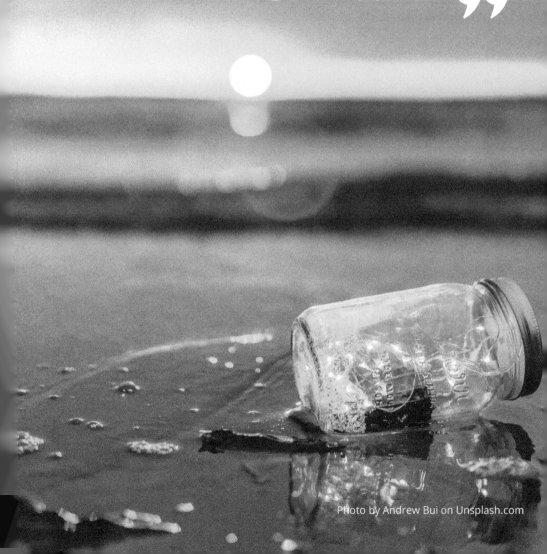

Feel how you will feel when you have already achieved it, and it will come into being. That's how the magic happens

A LETTER TO ANYONE STRUGGLING, INCLUDING MYSELF:

I knew I wanted to be a writer when I was very young. I entered a short story competition at school. I didn't win. Worse, I was bullied for even daring to think I was good enough to enter. Other kids called me horrid names because I was brought up in a caravan. People like me weren't allowed to dream big. A group of boys beat me up at school. I wasn't hurt, but I was terrified.

> It felt like the end of the world.

> But it wasn't.

I had a huge crush on a lad at school for ages. I sent him a Valentine's Day card. I was thrilled to get one in return – only to find the card I'd sent him ripped to shreds inside the envelope.

> It felt like the end of the world.

> But it wasn't.

My mum tried to hurt me.

> That felt like the end of the world.

> Luckily, it wasn't.

All the horrible things: my husband left me; I lost my job; I was badly injured in a car crash; my best friend stopped speaking to me; every one of the dozens and dozens of rejection letters for my writing; when my dad died; never having the baby I so desperately wanted; the pandemic—

> It all felt like the end of the world at the time.

> But it wasn't.

Many times, I've felt like ending it myself. A couple of times, I've tried.

> But it's not the end yet.

In the darkness, there is always light. If it's hard to see, we need to look with better eyes. In the morning, things shift and feel different. A smile, a hug, a purr, a sunny day, a "yes" – anything can make things just a little better.

Keep going. No matter how hard it may seem. Even if you feel it's the end of the world.

It is not the end.

Tina Baker,

author of #1 Kindle bestseller *Call Me Mummy.*

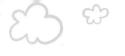

DEAR PAST VERSION OF ME,

I hope this letter finds you well.

I am writing to you today because my circumstances in the last year have radically transformed my life in many different ways. Or should I say *your* circumstances will change? I am your future self, here to warn you and reassure you everything will be just fine. Think of me as your guardian angel. Put your trust in me and the process you are about to go through.

If I could hand-deliver this letter to you, I would. To assure you the next few years will be a bumpy ride, but you will come out of the other side a much better version of yourself. You'll see, in time.

Right now, you are not living to your full potential – but don't worry, you will reach it. Trials and tribulations are just part of life. How can we transform into a better version of ourselves without struggle and hardship?

As I know you better than anyone else, I am aware you will want some evidence from me about future events which will unfold in our life. So, here goes.

Due to a mental breakdown, which happens due to exhaustion and work-related stress, you will have a lengthy recovery period. This also coincides with the threat of redundancy from your nine-year career. Listen to your body. It is pleading with you to please stop and rest. Do this! Rest until you feel you don't need to anymore.

You will be shattered into a million pieces, mentally and emotionally. I will be honest with you: following the struggle, you won't have much hope. But the people who love you the most will slowly help put you back together. Don't expect miracles. I know how impatient you are, but recovery doesn't happen overnight.

These two life-changing events will serve to make you realize what's important in life. You will decide to start living your purpose and following your dreams. It will no longer just sound like wonderful words people say. It will have meaning in your life, finally. You will feel a shift.

You will feel compelled to finally break the chains and share your story of living with anxiety for several years and hiding its impact very well. It's time to be free, so lift the weight off your shoulders. Don't expect anyone else to do it for you. Change comes from within.

You will start sharing your story to help other people in a similar situation, and you will be humbled to see the impact this is having on them. More importantly, the impact on those who don't contact you. It's helping them because they see someone openly talking about the horrible side of poor mental health, and they feel supported, less alone.

My dear, you will start to put measures in place never to return to a dark place in your mind or let anxiety rule your life. You control your thoughts now. You have the power to replace negative thoughts with positive ones. This will eventually turn into healthy habits. You learn to let negative emotions pass through without acting on them or allowing them to run wild in your mind.

I know you've had hopes and dreams all your life. Some of them you didn't chase because of anxiety, panic attacks, and lack of confidence. Some of them you did achieve, but it was excruciating to overcome the anxiety to complete the task. You achieved these dreams whilst wearing a mask and pretending you weren't living in fear. You are one strong woman to have lived life this way for so many years.

Have some open and honest conversations with those you love the most. They will understand. They always have done – you just didn't let them in.

I know you may find this letter daunting, but please know the struggle is vital for you to transform into a butterfly and change your life once and for all. No going back.

Don't run before you can walk. Take your recovery seriously. Your mind and body need you to be well so you can flourish in life. Listen to your inner voice. Learn to rest and recover every single day of your life from now on, to avoid ever experiencing this kind of burnout again. Self-care is vital, and you must practice it daily.

Value the most important things in life. Family, love, memories. Not working long days and getting no thanks for it. That's not life. That's plodding along.

By the end of this trauma, you will be full of hope. Something months back, you never thought you would achieve ever again.

This transformation will reassure you you're able to face any future life events or down periods head-on and get through them. You're building resilience, my love, and you're a fighter. But you don't need your future self to tell you that. You've always known.

Always listen to your intuition. It's got you through some tough times and can always be relied upon.

My advice is to take every opportunity thrown at you, flourish, and grow in confidence. Finally, do the job you've always wanted to do, helping others. But do it on your terms.

We only get one life, so let's both make it an amazing one. Create the life you want to live. What's stopping you?

I won't pretend this period of transformation is easy – it's far from it. But it will be amazing. Your outlook on life will completely change for the better.

Here's to your future self. I can't wait to meet the person you become on the other side of this. You were always destined for great things, you just didn't realize it yet. Everything in life has its time. This is your time to go out into the world and finally achieve your hopes and dreams.

With so much love,

Your Future Self

To ANYONE WHO NEEDS To PERSEVERE –

When I left university, I wrote to every radio station and television channel in Britain trying to find an opening, with a cassette radio reel for the radio stations.

Most didn't reply, but some radio stations did, saying that my letter and tape were "on file." It was only once I finally got a job in radio that I fully understood where they were filed: letters in the bin, cassettes re-used.

I also applied for the ITN Graduate Trainee scheme. I got an interview at which I majored on my love of foreign affairs and my desperate desire to cover foreign news. Unfortunately, they wanted someone who would specialize in industrial news and the Trade Unions!

I worked for a while covering Crown Court cases for local newspapers in London and Surrey, good training but very poorly paid.

Eventually I got a job at Metro Radio in Newcastle and later at Capital Radio in London.

I like to say that I eventually sneaked into ITN by the back door when no-one was looking, and spent ten very happy years there covering some of the biggest stories in the world before moving to Sky News.

Some years into my time at ITN, the Editor-in-Chief, Stewart Purvis, sent me a note with a copy of the shortlist for the Graduate trainee scheme all those years earlier with a hand-written note: "Perseverance pays."

Also, on that shortlist was someone else who wasn't taken on, my friend Ben Brown who went on to have a very successful career at BBC News.

So, I suppose the moral of the story is that, if you want something badly enough, just keep plugging away and you'll get there in the end.

Glen Ogazla

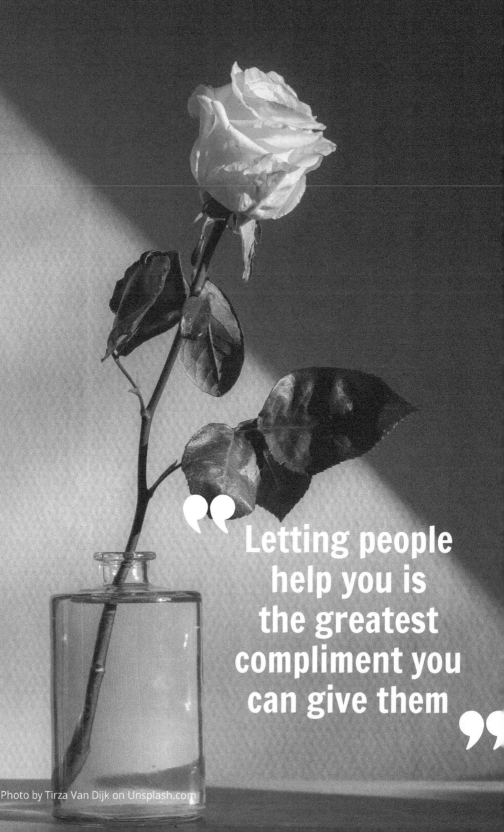

Letting people help you is the greatest compliment you can give them

DEAR NANNIE,

In search of adventure, you and your sister, both nurses, took the boat to England from Ireland in the 1930s. I can see you now on the top deck of the boat, laughing together at what was to come, as the wind whipped your auburn curls and the sharp breeze left a dew of salt on your faces.

When you arrived, London wasn't as welcoming as you expected. "No dogs, blacks or Irish" read signs on shop doors as the fear of difference reached deep into the heart of the city. Strong and determined, you kept your head down and worked hard, meeting the love of your life – a male nurse who was a talented saxophonist. Love and music lifted you, and soon you became part of a warm South London community. Sadly, the peace wasn't to last, and the country was at war.

During the Blitz, as the bombs rained down around you, rampaging London, you gave birth to a beautiful daughter with dark hair and bright blue eyes.

Despite the hardships, the three of you were a content little family, and 18 months later, you were expecting your second child. One night, your husband went to work at a nearby hospital. It wasn't his shift, but his friend wanted to swap shifts with him for a night, so he happily obliged. That night, a bomb razed the hospital to the ground, killing patients and medical workers, leaving you without a husband – and a toddler without her father.

> Every day, the little girl, barely three years old, would look out of the window, waiting for him to come home - to walk up the path as always, catch sight of her and smile, his eyes crinkling with delight. But he never did.

Now you were a young widow with another baby on the way, facing financial hardship and the stigma of being a single mother in 1940s England. The kindness of strangers was to save you. Your children never went without at Christmas – you hand-sewed exquisite dresses for your daughter, while neighbors gave toys to your newborn son, brought you home-cooked meals with what little rations they had.

Love, kindness and support embraced you, and you were not too proud to accept it. Years later, when your daughter – my mother – nursed you through cancer in the final months of your life, she felt honored to be able to return the love you never failed to show her.

Sadly, I never met you. You lost your battle with cancer just before I was born. But we remember you and our brave grandfather, who stepped in to help his friend without question.

It takes courage to ask for help and even greater courage to accept it. It is not a weakness but a strength. People are kind and loyal, and good. Letting them help you is the greatest compliment you can give them.

Love,

Anne Amlot

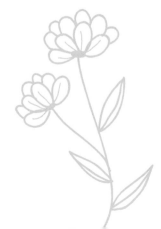

TO ANYONE RUNNING FROM THEIR PAIN –

May we turn and face up to what causes us discomfort; may we stand strong in times of great challenge and struggle because we have weathered the storms and chaos within.

May life be an ever-unfolding of gracious acceptance and finding an ever-evolving path of deep love, compassion and care towards ourselves.

When we run away from, try to disengage, find ways to disassociate and turn away from our pain, our wounds, our sorrow, our confusion, our struggles, our anger… it only ever grows into deeper lesions.

> Because your pain and suffering are your gateway to freedom.

It is the one-way ticket to great transformation and healing. The track gets very rough at points, but the journey is magical, no doubt.

Do not see the pain and struggle as something to avoid or fear – no, it is quite the opposite. On the other side lies your greatest and most powerful self.

Running away won't give you closure; closure will. Hiding, dismissing, ignoring won't bring you healing; facing it, embracing it and saying, "let's do this" will.

Life is always giving us the chance to grow, to experience better, to step up and really LIVE!

"I can't be bothered" won't do anything but keep you stuck in a perpetual loop of stagnation and frustration. We just have to muster the energy and accept the challenge or stay the same and probably complain about it.

It's all a choice. Go after what lights you up.

Anonymous

TO ANYONE WHO WANTS TO BELIEVE AND ACHIEVE –

Hello, everyone, my name is Pamerjit, and I'm a 49-year-old female.

I hope you enjoy reading my letter and you gain something from it.

I have four sisters and three brothers. I am Indian-Sikh.

When I was growing up, we really never had much money or toys but we did have love for each other. My mum taught us great manners and my dad taught us how to save money, which I have passed onto my daughter India, aged nine.

My dad was a door-to-door salesman, and my mum was a busy housewife and everything else that went with this role.

At school, I wasn't good at reading, writing or math, but I had a great heart and loved making people smile.

I would get extra English in Primary School and the teacher was AMAZING, but at High School the teacher didn't really care about us in her small cold room, which was hidden away in the corner. I used to hate going there and was very embarrassed as the other children knew.

I had to work twice as hard to achieve my qualifications in sports and in childcare.

> I made a promise with myself that if I ever had
> a child, I would not let them suffer as I did
> with English at school.

I made sure that when my daughter, India, was very young, around 3 months, I would read to her every day and show her pictures.

Today she can read, write and spell much better than I ever could. I am so happy that she will not suffer the way I did. (No child should.)

They said I was dyslexic at school but never tested.

At high school, I developed a passion for sports. I was really good at all sports, but my favorites were hockey and running, as I discovered after running the 800 meters at school. I nearly came first but ended up fourth or fifth as the girl who ran at a running club always came first. I nearly killed myself as I had never ever ran this distance in my life.

As we never had much money, and coming from a large Asian family, I never joined the hockey club or running club.

Also, in those days, Asians, especially girls, were never seen or encouraged to do any kind of sports. My mum would encourage us to do any sport we could if it was available through the school. Nowadays, it's still very rare to see Asians in sport unless it's cricket.

When Covid hit, the gyms were closed. I have over 25 years' experience running on the treadmill. This is where I did all my running, having never lost the passion that came from that 800 meter run at school.

I still wanted to run so I was forced out of my comfort zone to run outside, which I didn't like as I have a love-hate relationship with this. I didn't think I could do it – it felt unsafe, plus where I lived was all new to me. I was unsure – could I actually take this challenge on? It was really scary to me.

I started off with a slow pace, time and distance. As I say, all this was much easier for me on a treadmill, where I would do speed work and long distance running. Outside, it was all new to me, but I was going to give it a go. I did this four to five times a week. One day, I fell outside, but I was determined to keep going. I came home, cleaned myself up, got straight back out there and ran eight miles. Even though my knees were cut and bleeding, and my hands were badly grazed, bleeding and sore, I still never gave up.

I ran my first Virtual London Marathon in 2020. The time was 3 hours 44 minutes and 47 seconds. In my head, I was just thinking, "Believe and achieve and I will do it it!"

In 2020, I ran nine virtual marathons on my own (except for my first ever Virtual London Marathon, as I had my daughter, her dad and a few friends cheering me on), and a further 20 marathons in 2021, two of which were live.

Not bad for someone who just ran on a treadmill and still does.

My siblings and I lost both parents in India at different times on the same day. I was only 20 then and never got to say goodbye to them at the funeral.

We never let this experience stop us from achieving what we wanted to do in life. I was determined to live my life as much as I could the way I wanted to.

You cannot let your upbringing, lack of money, ethnicity and others get in your way of any opportunities. Only you get to dictate how you can achieve amazing opportunities and goals within your life.

Take every opportunity given to you and never be afraid to try something new as long as you are safe and happy to do so.

Never ever give up on your dreams.

If you have a passion inside you, PLEASE follow it through if it's possible to do so.

Try not to let negative thoughts talk you out of doing things.

You've got this.

Grab every opportunity that comes your way.

I have told my young daughter, India, that she can do anything and achieve anything if she puts her mind to it.

My motto in life is "Believe and achieve."

NOW go out there and achieve your dreams.

Good luck everyone.

Love, live, laugh and enjoy life to the full.

Love,

Pamerjit x

Try not to let negative thoughts talk you out of doing things.
YOU'VE GOT THIS

My moto in life is Believe and Achieve.

NOW go out there and Achieve your Dreams.

Goodluck Everyone.

Love, Live, Laugh & enjoy life to the full.

Love

Pamerjit x

DEAR YOUNGER SELF,

It feels hard, doesn't it? Conforming to the norms that have been set for you. You don't need to let go of those dreams that keep your mind whizzing at night.

Dreams aren't just for sleeping. They are sneak peeks of what is yet to come. Although it's difficult to walk through a busy crowd that's walking against you, keep pushing, keep striving because the best is yet to come.

I believe. That's all that matters.

Love, your grateful future self

Alicia Thompson

Dreams aren't just for sleeping. They are sneak peeks of what is yet to come

Believe

To Anyone with a Creative Spirit –

From an early age, I was an energetic and curious child. And even though I suffered hardships and pain in my life, I never lost my energy or curiosity.

I was born at *La Casa Azul* (the Blue House), a house my father had built. My father was a talented and successful photographer, and the Mexican government commissioned him to photograph the historical buildings and landscapes of Mexico. I loved looking at my father's photos. They taught me about Mexican architecture, art and history. They made me proud of my country and my heritage. When my father wasn't busy taking photographs, he liked to paint. Sometimes he took me with him when he went to the countryside to use his paints and brushes. I loved watching my father create images on the canvas.

When I was six years old, I contracted polio. It was so serious that I needed to stay in my bed for almost nine months. It was very difficult for someone as curious and energetic as me to be stuck in bed. The polio left my right leg weak and thin, but that didn't stop me from playing football, wrestling, boxing and swimming. I was determined not to let my illness stop me from being me. The kids in my neighborhood called me *pata de palo*, which means "peg leg," so as I got older, I wore trousers, long dresses and skirts to hide my leg. I didn't want anyone to know I was different, make fun of me, or feel sorry for me.

Even though I had missed a lot of school, I was admitted to *Escuela Nacional Preparatoria* (National Preparatory School), in Mexico City – the best high school in the country. There were 2,000 boys and only 35 girls, but I wasn't scared or nervous. I was excited about being away from home and meeting new people. The friends I made, the things we talked about and what I learned in class, changed my life. My favorite classes were science and math, and I decided I wanted to be a doctor. One day a famous artist named Diego Rivera came to our school. After the Mexican Revolution, the government had chosen him as one of the artists to paint murals throughout the country, to help Mexicans understand their past, make them proud of their country, and give them hope for the future. Even though Diego was famous, I called him names and put soap on the stairs to see if he would slip and fall.

One day, as my friend Alejandro and I were on our way home from school, the bus we were riding in was hit by a trolley car. I suffered horrible injuries – the metal arm from one of the bus seats had gone through my body. At first the doctors weren't sure that I would survive. As I lay in that hospital bed, I thought about how I might have died. The memories of that day would stay with me for the rest of my life. But I was a strong and determined person. I had overcome polio, and I would not let this accident keep me from living the life I wanted for myself.

Finally, I was strong enough to go home. However, I was still in a full-body plaster cast. I couldn't move or sit up, but I needed something to do. I asked my father if I could borrow his paints. My mother had a carpenter make a special easel so that I could paint while I was lying on my back. A large mirror was hung over my bed so that I could look at myself as I painted. The pictures I painted included religious symbols and Mexican folk-art. I also painted many self-portraits, because I was so often alone and because I am the subject I know best.

> Painting allowed me to forget my pain. I decided I no longer wanted to be a doctor, I wanted to be an artist.

Once I recovered, I was happy to see my friends again. Guess who was at one of the parties I went to? Diego Rivera! He didn't remember me, but I remembered him. A few days after the party, I got up the nerve to ask him to look at four of my paintings. He wasn't that impressed with three of them, but he really liked one of them. He said the painting was original and that I had talent. After that, Diego and I started to spend a lot of time together. We were falling in love. I also knew Diego would be a great teacher if I wanted to be a painter. We were a bit of an odd couple, but eventually we married in 1929. After Diego and I were married, I didn't paint very much. Looking after Diego, a world-famous artist, was a full-time job. This frustrated me, but I didn't say anything to my husband.

In 1930, Diego was asked to work in the US, and I went with him. Although we went to fabulous parties and met lots of people, I was often alone, because Diego was working most of the time. I finally decided it was time to pick up my paintbrushes and start painting again. My paintings revealed how much I missed Mexico, my discomfort about being in the

US, and the suffering of people during the Great Depression. I wanted my art to communicate that, whilst I was physically in the US, my body and soul were still in Mexico.

After three long years in the US, Diego and I moved back to Mexico. We had begun to argue while in the US, and our fights became more frequent and louder once we were back home. The energy and emotion I felt at this time went into my paintings. It was during these difficult times that many people said I created my best and most interesting paintings. Even though my personal life was difficult, I was becoming more successful as an artist and more people started noticing my work. My paintings weren't always easy to look at, but they made people think and feel. I finally felt that people were seeing Frida Kahlo, not the wife of Diego Rivera.

Things between Diego and me became even more strained. We respected each other as artists, but being husband and wife was too hard. We ultimately decided to divorce in 1939.

After our divorce, my career took off. I had exhibitions in New York City and San Francisco. While I was in San Francisco, Diego came to see me. We truly missed each other and decided to give marriage another try. We moved back to the Blue House, and I was thrilled and comforted by the fact that my childhood home would be my studio. In 1953, I was finally given my first solo show in Mexico. I'd had solo shows in other countries, but to have one in my own country made me so proud. At this point, my body was starting to let me down, and my doctor said I shouldn't go to the show, but I didn't listen. I had my four-poster bed set up in the gallery and I laid there as people viewed my work. It was almost as if I was a work of art myself.

Even though I had a strong will, my body was weak, and each day became more of a struggle. One of the last paintings I created contained the words, *viva la vida*. In English that means 'long live life'. My life was full of pain and heartache; however, I was determined to always keep those words in my head and in my heart. No matter what was in my path, I wanted to live life on my own terms.

No te rindas!

Frida

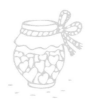

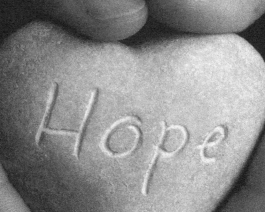

To ANYONE WHO NEEDS HOPE –

In June 2009, at the age of 33 and a single parent of three young children, I joined Lothian and Borders Police as a Police Constable. L & B was one of eight police forces within Scotland, independent of each other. On 1st April 2013, all eight police forces joined together and became Police Scotland.

Throughout my career I was a competent and dedicated officer with strong ambitions and believed it to be my future. I was passionate about obtaining justice for the vulnerable and protecting others from harm. I truly loved my job.

In 2016, I successfully completed a firearms course; it was extremely liberating, and I was proud to have achieved success in such a difficult area. I became an authorized firearms officer based in Edinburgh. At that time only 3% of firearms officers were female.

> I rode the wave of accomplishment and pride for what seemed like forever, my confidence and commitment to the job was evident and I was held in high regard.

I was enthusiastic, driven, joyful and fulfilled. I believe these character traits positively influenced others around me. I built what I believed to have been strong relationships with fellow officers; the camaraderie gave me an overwhelming sense of acceptance and belonging. My trust in Police Scotland and that of my colleagues was unquestionable.

Unfortunately, this love for life and the enjoyment I got from my career changed. From May 2017, I experienced misogyny, discrimination, bullying and harassment from senior male and female officers. Although I had once been a very confident and strong female, I found that over a period of a few months, this had started to dissipate. Unlike any other division or career that I had experienced, I found the Firearms division to be extremely archaic, shrouded in secrecy and controlling.

In January 2018, I received an email from my temporary Inspector forbidding me from working with another female officer, and his reason for this was due to our physical capabilities and to balance out testosterone. The email was not only offensive, discriminatory and a misuse of his authority, but it was the cherry on top for me. In less than a year I had been victimized by this man and others beyond comprehension, I was even accused of gross misconduct by another temporary Inspector – he accused me of throwing my utility belt which had a loaded gun on it. This never happened.

Following the submission of my complaint, I was victimized by management and my perpetrators were promoted to substantive Inspectors. It was clear that management did not want to acknowledge there was a problem and wanted rid of me. My colleagues, who had once been very supported and encouraging, abandoned me. I felt betrayed. These officers started to express their disapproval, sighting me as a drama queen, and that by submitting a complaint I had taken it too far. I believe management's response to nurture bad behavior left these officers feeling threatened and in fear of reprisals; the result was self-preservation and victim blaming. My perpetrators appeared to have been absolved of any wrongdoing and I was identified as the problem.

I was devastated, I felt alone and when I went home would be inconsolable with grief. I had no choice; I left the job I loved. Being in an environment where I felt unwanted and suppressed was causing me to become extremely unhappy. I felt fearful of my colleagues whose integrity, values and ethics I now questioned; I was no longer a jovial or confident individual. My character and personality were changing. I felt in a state of chaos and confusion. I felt unsupported and discarded.

I was prevented from speaking out for a long time due to being a police officer (regulations are in place to prevent this) and could not find others who had experienced the same or similar. I faced many obstructions, mainly from the very departments who were meant to help and support me. I was misled by HR (human resources) and only provided limited information around the grievance procedure. I soon established that there were other women who had been through the same experience but had signed NDAs, (non-disclosure agreements); they had been silenced.

I had provided justice to many people over my police career and yet I could not get it within the organization when I sought it out. I was left with no choice; I took legal action against Police Scotland in July 2018 and retired due to ill health in April 2020. I refused to accept a payout or sign an NDA because I knew there were others like me. I did not want to be complicit in their suppression of inequality and felt a duty to bring awareness and light to this situation because without it there would be no change.

In November 2020, I went public. I now share my journey with the world. I believe NDAs to be oppressive to women's equity. My hope is to educate and bring awareness to inequality, social injustice and the abuse of power and authority within Police Scotland. I did not have a choice; this was my final duty as a Police Officer, one I take great pride in.

In October 2021, I obtained acknowledgment and accountability through an employment tribunal. My victimization case was upheld in its entirety and there have now been calls from the Scottish government and the Chief Constable of Police Scotland for an independent review of my case and the use of NDAs by public bodies.

My health has slowly improved. I know that the deterioration in my mental health was and still is directly related to being discriminated against, victimized, and being prevented from talking about my situation with others. I have now found many other women in the same situation and through talking and sharing, I truly believe equality for women can be achieved, we just need more of us to do it. We need others to make a stand to evoke change.

I have faith that this gives you hope and encouragement that every one of us can evoke change.

This journey took my career, affected my mental health, and impacted me and my family significantly over four years. However, the feeling of accomplishment, acknowledgment and accountability is phenomenal. To have done nothing would have made me complicit in their behavior and a hypocrite. I now live life very differently and far better than I ever did. I would not change a thing.

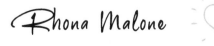

Rhona Malone

To ANYONE NEEDING TO INVEST IN THEMSELVES –

If your heart feels like it's breaking

And your body's filled with dread,

If your head feels like it's racing

And you'd rather stay in bed

If talking is a challenge

And you'd rather hide away

Take time to remember

Things won't always be this way.

If each breath feels like hard labor

And each step you take a chore,

It's ok to take some time out

Until you feel yourself once more.

Try to focus on the little things

That bring to you a smile

Investing in your mental health

and wellbeing is worthwhile.

Sarah Mullin

TO ANYONE LOOKING FOR HOPE AND BELIEF –

Growing up, I always knew what I wanted to do. That was to create "art." I'd paint, play an instrument, and write stories. I've always expressed myself creatively, and the people around me didn't always champion that. But that was okay, because deep inside myself, I knew I was an artist and that the only way I would truly be happy, be free, was to create something that I was proud of.

> My biggest love has always been writing. "I'm going to be an author," I'd say at ten. A couple of the adults around me were encouraging, most weren't. They wanted me to be something I wasn't, to pick a different career.

I'd be lying if I said that this didn't cause me to doubt my choices. I was a very average student most of my life. I wasn't the sort of student most teachers praised, or thought would do something amazing in life. I kind of just glided through my studies. For my GCSE's I picked subjects that had a broad range of careers like graphic design and ICT. In sixth form, I studied Graphic Design and Media Studies. In university, I studied advertising because there were a lot of job opportunities in that field.

However, it wasn't until I graduated that I really felt lost. *What was I going to do now*? I thought. I knew by my second year that working in advertising wasn't a career I truly wanted.

Then in Ramadan 2018, my life changed … and it all started with an idea for a book. I spent the next nine months writing it and then sent it into competitions where I heard nothing back (no surprise now, because looking back, it wasn't very good). The rejection was painful, but I moved on to the next idea. This was a longer book, and I spent two whole months planning it before I even wrote a word. I then worked on that for an entire year before entering it into a competition. I didn't get my hopes up this time because I knew, even if I was rejected again, I would keep going with another idea. To my surprise, I didn't get rejected this time, but was awarded a prize by a huge publishing company.

I then wrote the beginning of two more books, which got me a lot of attention, agents asking to see more of my work because they could "see something" in my writing.

All these things felt amazing, but nothing felt better than knowing that it all happened because I believed in myself. I kept going, even in the face of rejection. And I would be lying if I said I still don't get rejected today for things, because I do. But because I have myself on my side, I know I will make my dream come true, *In Shaa Allah*.

> I believe we are not burdened with problems
> that we cannot overcome. We are only as good
> as our belief in ourselves.

I'm still not at the point I want to be. My dream is to be a published author. But I'm closer to that goal than I was last month, last week, even yesterday. I know that this is a journey and there is no real "destination." There are bumps and potholes along the way but hope and self-belief keep me going. I'm further than I've ever been, and tomorrow I'll be even further.

So, if there is anything that I'd say to young people, it's keep going. Don't look for outside validation because it may not come. Look within yourself. Know that your dreams and hopes are valid and that only you can make them come true. There might be a lot of hard times, or maybe you're a lucky person and things fall into place quickly. But all that really matters is that you keep going, keep dedicating time to whatever you are passionate about and I'm sure one day you will be sitting in a comfortable chair, looking back at how far you've come, feeling proud of yourself for never giving up.

With my words, I create art. What will you create?

H. Jama

"With my words I create art. What will you create?"

To ANYONE FACING CHALLENGES –

Growing up, I always had a vision of how my life would look at different milestones – how it would look when I finished school, started university, graduated and then entered the working world. Although I knew that an individual's dreams were susceptible to change, I just didn't ever entertain that mine might also change its course.

Looking back, I realize it was because I was afraid of being open to experiences and opportunities, to self-discovery, and I feared change because of how I defined it. I didn't allow myself to see past the life I thought I would have, because being in the familiar is always more comforting than being in the unknown. Realizing this, it isn't hard to understand why I felt "safer" in the familiar reality of difficulty and hardship, then in the unknown reality of defying the odds, as I experienced what seemed like challenge after challenge in my late teens.

Fast forward five years, I know what I would tell that younger version of me if I could talk to her. The first thing I would remind her of is her power.

Each of us are uniquely powerful individuals,
with the capacity to do better, strive for more,
and achieve our dreams.

When we reach a hurdle in the road, the two paths ahead will either be a path we follow where we realize our power to overcome the hurdle, or a path where we surrender to a situation because we have interpreted it as impossible to move past. It is at these times that we must battle our intrusive thoughts and choose to own our power.

We must remind ourselves that we have everything we need to overcome challenges inside of us. There is no age, no background, no limitation that can hold us back. Once we realize this, the rest will come naturally if we trust it will.

The second thing I would tell her is that the meaning we give the things that we experience in our lives can make all the difference between overcoming adversity or not. Everything that happens in life is neutral, but it is the meaning we give these experiences that determines our reaction to them. When challenges occur, understanding that you will be wiser, stronger and more resilient once you overcome them is how you redefine what can be perceived as only a negative event. I would urge the younger version of me to be brave in the pursuit of her goals. In order to experience a new reality, we must think new thoughts and do new things. In order to overcome challenges, we must be brave enough to think beyond our current situations and to take action. Inaction can be more damaging than we think, and we must not let fear hold us back.

One of the most important pieces of advice I would give her would be to always look forward, unless you are learning from the past. Do not let your past define you, because all your past is a series of old thoughts, behaviors and actions that led to experiences. Your future is defined by what you do in the present, and it is the positive attitude of knowing that things can get better that will allow your mind to free itself from the attachment of your past experiences. Visualizing what it is like to be on the other side of your hardship will assist you in overcoming it because we believe what we can see.

My experience of adversity has taught me lessons as well as helped to mold me into the person I am today. Since what felt like a really difficult time in my life, I have gone from strength to strength, working towards my goals and living a life I am creating. If I experience a challenge, as we all do in its various forms, I trust that I have it within me, within those around me, to overcome it. I have given myself permission to forgive, to learn, to evolve. If it wasn't for the challenges I faced, I don't know how long it would have taken me to develop the skills, knowledge and experience to aim higher.

Adversity has taught me that the potential to feel better and do better is always there – it is up to us to align to it and to chase it. Owning the unique experiences which make you who you are, and knowing that you are the creator of your life will set you free to overcome adversity and to thrive.

Jaya Pathak

Co-Executive Director at Yet Again UK

To ANYONE WHO FEELS THEY'VE FAILED –

Sometimes, you apply for a job in hope more than expectation, knowing it's probably not going to come off. Sometimes, you know you've got a decent chance, as long as you do everything right, but sometimes – well, sometimes you instinctively know that this is a job with your name written on it, that you're not so much applying for a job as fulfilling your destiny.

I remember being in that situation. I'd been appointed as a Deputy Head a year earlier, but after two weeks settling into the new school, my Headteacher went off on sick leave, which eventually became retirement.

The next four terms were challenging but exhilarating as I threw myself into the role. Pupils and parents seemed to like me, staff were supportive and every governor's meeting ended with a word of thanks and the comment, "What on earth would we have done if Paul hadn't been here?"

Finally, the job was advertised. I spent a long time on my application and made sure my preparation was just right. The day before the interview, I received a card from the staff wishing me luck, and lost count of the number of parents who told me that I was a shoe-in.

There was only one other candidate, a Head from a local school. Everything went well. My presentation was a thing of beauty, my prepared answers slick. I could reference everything I'd accomplished over the past year and show off my detailed knowledge of the school. I went home, rang my wife with an update, and awaited the phone call.

You're probably one step ahead. The phone call came. They thanked me for everything I'd done for the school, congratulated me on my performance during the day … and told me the job had gone to the other candidate.

I couldn't tell you the reasons – I was in no state of mind to listen. I mumbled a "thanks for letting me know" and hung up. I sat there feeling numb and was still in the same chair when my wife came in an hour later with a bottle of wine, ready for a celebration which never happened.

I didn't react well. I felt cheated, that I'd been lied to. They had taken advantage of me, strung me along while I had kept the school going, only to ditch me at the first opportunity. The next day was hard, I was the victim of my own hubris, but I fronted it out and thanked everyone for their support, all the while dreading the next few weeks during which I would still be the Acting Headteacher – good enough to be the caretaker, but not good enough to be trusted with the job permanently. I resolved to stick around for just long enough to be able to apply for a job without my application looking like a fit of pique.

As it happened, I stayed for two more years. The new Headteacher arrived, and made her presence felt straight away. The office, which had been unchanged in a year apart from a small photo of my wedding and a framed picture of Goodison Park was now resplendent with dried flowers and potpourri, and inspirational quotes framed on the wall.

Her initial Assembly was brilliant – warm, authoritative, funny – and set the tone for her first few weeks. She suggested we write a School Development Plan together and involved me in every step. A decent start then, in her first few weeks of doing my job.

Over the next two years I watched her at close quarters. She asked people's opinions, considered them, but was unafraid to make decisions. She had a way of passing on difficult messages supportively and professionally, in a way that didn't really brook any argument. She was thorough, hardworking, knowledgeable and always professional. The school grew and blossomed under her leadership. Ofsted came and liked what they saw.

She was also kind and took an interest in people. She was particularly kind to me and instinctively knew that she was dealing with someone with a bruised and fragile ego. She had a way of giving me good advice whilst at the same time making it sound like she was asking my opinion, and without realizing it, I was learning my trade every day. It was my Head Teacher apprenticeship.

Eventually, I felt I was ready, and applied for headships. The first one I didn't get, up against a strong and well-respected internal candidate. The second one was different – I knew I had a chance and it felt like a good fit.

There was a moment in the final interview when they asked me, "What makes you think you are ready to be a Headteacher?" I can't remember my answer, probably a fairly cliched response. However, I do remember it as a moment of clarity. I couldn't be certain that I was ready, but I was absolutely certain that I hadn't been ready two years earlier.

I had learnt because there were people who were prepared to make the right decision, even though it was not the one I wanted. In that in the moment of disappointment it's hard to see the bigger picture, and the job that is the perfect fit for each of us is by definition the one we eventually get.

In the meantime, every application and interview really is a learning experience.

As Henry Ford said, "Failure is simply the opportunity to begin again, this time more intelligently." It just sometimes takes time to realize it.

Paul

To Anyone Who Feels Helpless,

I find sometimes that everything going on in the world feels so negative. Every day in the media there is another story about a terrorist attack, someone else who has been murdered, another warning about the damage we are doing to the planet. It just feels so all encompassing; social media is full of people who have perfect lives and bodies and still seem to be able to eat chocolate at the same time!

Working in the police sadly magnifies the negative feeling; on an operational basis you tend to be involved in murders and other serious incidents; you try to help but usually the harm is already done. You see children born into certain social situations and you realize the lack of chances that they will have and how the chances are they will end up in a life of crime.

Then there are the things that really hurt: the issues around a lack of police action initially to the child exploitation scandal and more recently the tragic and horrific murder of Sarah Everard.

Sometimes working for an organization at times that everyone seems to hate can be so hard. But I speak for myself and colleagues when I say most officers joined for the right reasons: to help the public, to protect people and to better people's lives.

I used to find this feeling of helplessness, thinking, "What could I, as just one human being, do to affect any of this?" It felt like all the power to change the big issues lay with world leaders and politicians and I, just merely one individual, didn't have the power to change anything.

Then I remember the poem that my mum wrote in my 21st birthday card.

Once upon a time, there was an old man who used to go to the ocean for exercise.

One day, the old man was walking along a beach that was littered with thousands of starfish that had been washed ashore by the high tide. As he walked, he came upon a young boy who was eagerly throwing the starfish back into the ocean, one by one.

Puzzled, the man looked at the boy and asked what he was doing.

The young boy paused, looked up, and replied, "Throwing starfish into the ocean. The tide has washed them up onto the beach and they can't return to the sea by themselves. When the sun gets high, they will die, unless I throw them back into the water."

The old man replied, "But there must be tens of thousands of starfish on this beach. I'm afraid you won't really be able to make much of a difference."

The boy bent down, picked up yet another starfish and threw it as far as he could into the ocean. Then he turned, smiled, and said, "It made a difference to that one!"

And that, I have found, is the trick to managing all that feeling of not being able to affect anything. It's helping that one starfish. For me, it started as a younger child baking cookies for the ChildLine cookie challenge, probably only raising £20, but maybe it was that £20 that was the call that made a difference. Abseiling down Manchester United with Fred the Red at 16 (did I mention I don't like football)!! Carrying on the craziness at university to raise a good number for different local, regional and national charities though various crazy ways! Hitchhiking from Durham to Dublin in a farmer's van with a load of sheep – my favorite experience! I always, if I have time, buy a homeless person a meal and listen to their life story.

More recently, whilst fundraising has taken me to some amazing places from the Durham University duck race to the Queen's garden party, I have learnt that I prefer the personal approach – it lets me know I am making a difference. So, I volunteer for Barnardos as the independent visitor for a child in care. This has been my favorite volunteer journey to date. Every few weeks, I take my nominated lovely child out to crazy

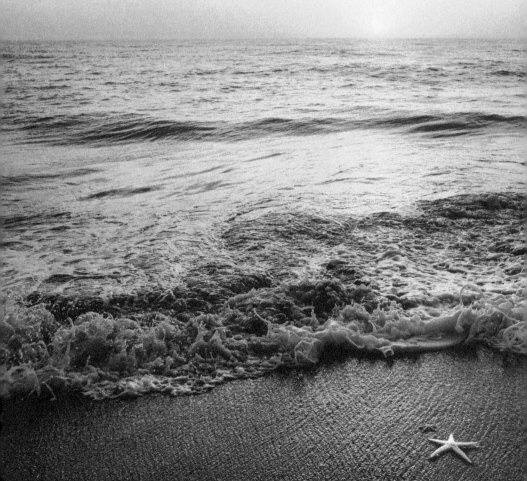

The whole world
can be changed, one
starfish at a time

Photo by Todd Trapanin Unsplash.com

golf, ten pin bowling or even to the football! She is one child in a family of ten and loves the time on her own. I have also worked hard to get her younger brother a mentor as he doesn't go to school and is only eight.

> My ethos of my letter to you is very much centered around changing one starfish at a time.

The coffee you buy the homeless person, the time you give to a charity … the whole can be changed, one starfish at a time.

It doesn't need to be a big gesture like raising money for a charity. It's the little things that matter – giving your chair up for the elderly person on the train or volunteering for that project you haven't got the time for.

So, stand on your beach and throw that starfish back in.

Tasha Evans

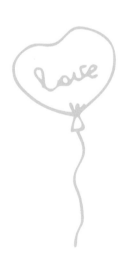

TO ANYONE WHO NEEDS TO HEAR THIS –

When I was sixteen years old, I got a tattoo on my back. I was young and naïve but, even then, I realized the importance of getting a tattoo that *really* meant something. One that represented a philosophy which I could carry forward for the rest of my life. At the end of the day, I was going to be stuck with this damn thing, so it might as well be something important!

I settled on the yin-yang symbol. To the ancient Chinese, it represented the interconnected and counterbalancing forces of the entire universe. To me, it represented the eternal balance of happiness and sadness, good and bad, right and wrong.

It helped me realize one of the most important lessons I have ever learned: a little bad can be found in all good things but, just as important (if not more so), a little good can be found in all bad things. As a child who was bullied at school, being able to find the light in dark times was fundamental to driving me forward. To put on my uniform and walk through those school gates knowing the bullies, and the dark times, would be there waiting for me.

Those bad times eventually passed. I changed schools, made new friends and was happy. Happier, in fact, than any other child in my class because I was finally free from the bullying I had endured. If I could go back in time, I wouldn't change a thing because that bullying strengthened me. I am the person I am today because of it.

Fast forward almost three decades. The year is 2020. I am now 36 years of age. I have a wonderful wife, two fantastic children, a lovely pet dog and a nice home. Things are good. But the tattoo on my back is about to deliver a powerful reminder of what it represents.

It was the end of the August bank holiday weekend, and I woke up feeling groggy, like I was hungover, although I had only had a glass of wine the night before. What ensued was two weeks of the most profound agony I have ever experienced. Searing, relentless pain in my ear, jaw and eye, all localized to the left side of my head.

During those hard weeks, I would pump myself full of powerful painkillers

> **A little bad can be found in all good things but, just as importantly, a little good can be found IN ALL BAD THINGS**

and sleep during the day. At night, when the painkillers had worn off, I would lie awake, grinding my teeth in pain, sometimes resorting to crawling around on the floor like an animal, because staying still was unbearable.

I was in and out of hospital, given more drugs, and had a full suite of blood tests. When they came back clean, I had MRI, CAT and EKG scans and an audio assessment. Everything came back inconclusive. I saw a few specialists who couldn't put their finger on the issue. As time passed, the painful side of the illness subsided, but it left me with tinnitus in my left ear, extreme fatigue, and balance issues. I was a stone lighter than I had been two weeks earlier.

Eventually I was diagnosed with a vestibular disorder, although the cause was, and continues to be, unknown. The specialists prescribed me various new drugs, including anti-epilepsy medicine designed to suppress abnormal brain activity. When this didn't work, I tried mindfulness, meditation and even went as far as visiting a hyperbaric chamber, but nothing worked.

This went on for many months. I couldn't play football with my son. I couldn't pick up my daughter for fear of dropping her. I couldn't walk up the stairs without gripping the handrail tightly. A ten-minute walk outside exhausted me to the point of collapse. I worried about what my wife would think of me. I felt ashamed that if something happened to my family while we were out, I would be in no position to protect them. I felt more vulnerable than I had ever felt in my life. I felt pathetic.

Sticking with my philosophy, I decided to find the light in the dark. I started writing.

As well as being one of my biggest passions, writing was something which I could do without discomfort. It enabled me to forget my troubles both physically and psychologically. Before long, I started to feel like I was doing what I was *meant* to be doing. As time passed, I started to recover. I saw a physio and he set out a regime of visual and movement exercises designed to challenge me. They were hard work, but that was the point. As time progressed, the symptoms eased, albeit very slowly.

Fast forward a year and I am now a published author of four books, with a fifth on the way. I am quite literally doing my dream job. A step I never would have taken if it hadn't been for the illness. As for my health, I am pleased to report that I am 95% recovered. While elements still linger, I can now drive a car, play football with my son, pick up my daughter and swing her around (although she's getting rather heavy for that).

I am now a full-time writer. Is it all sunshine and roses? No. Writing is hard work and, as with any profession, there are downsides. As with the yin-yang, there is always that little bit of bad in the good.

So, if you're reading this letter and life is going really well, then enjoy it. Savor every moment. You can use these memories as a beacon of hope when the bad times come.

If you're reading this letter and you are going through a tough time, then try to find that little bit of light, the good. It's there somewhere, I promise. Grab onto it. Let it carry you through the darkness, because you'll come out on the other side soon.

Yours,

Matt Whelan

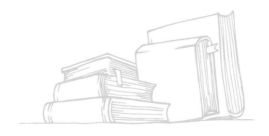

DEAR 16-YEAR-OLD ME,

Nobody in your family has been to uni. Your older siblings aren't into study, don't swat for exams.

But you're different, a little out of step with the hubbub of the world. A reader, writer, thinker. When you look at books, a shy thought floats in. *I'd like to see my name on one of those.* It's barely an ambition you can acknowledge as frail as a bubble, and as easily popped.

Your teachers see the bubble. They keep it alive. They tell you, *aim high.*

Really high.

You start to hear the word "Oxbridge" bandied about. You find out, too late to escape ridicule, that it's Oxford and Cambridge mixed together. Doubty Gremlin squats on your shoulder and says - *What? Not you. You're not clever, not like that.*

But, you dare to believe. You believe you can get those grades. You come from a state school, with no record of students accepted into the top unis. There's no extra support on offer. But you read the extra books. You go the extra mile. You get your head down.

Apply to one of the colleges on the outskirts of Oxford, is the advice. *You've got more chance there.*

The big interview doesn't go well. You're overawed, out of your depth, too nervous to think straight. Your name is chalked up on the board – rejected here, but another college'll take a look … A central college, with stone columns and squares of grass you can't walk on. The interview is slated for 10pm – in a dark study where three tired dons sink backwards into old wingback armchairs with hands steepled. It goes terribly, and Doubty Gremlin cackles in delight.

But an offer comes, by letter – and it feels like some kind of mistake? Your parents jump and shriek. They start to eye you a little differently, as if you're an out-of-control firework, streaking off to *God Knows Where. Where does she get her brains?*

Hell, you're on your way.

Oxford is a shock. You're homesick, the work is hard – dozens of books to speed read a week, in far flung libraries spread around the city. But you wear self-discipline like an old coat cinched in at the waist, and you treat it like a working day: 9-5pm for historical study. Then, party time. *Work Hard, Play Hard*.

First year exams – you get a first.

Third year exams – you get another first, one of the highest.

That's a double first.

Stay here, they say, *study more*, but no, you're done with that.

There's a world out there.

Except, the world doesn't want to know. Who cares about your double first in history? Where's your work experience? How to explain that you've been too busy studying for that …

So, you doss down on friend's sofas and work for FREE. On the local paper. For weeks. Collecting those by-lines. Learning how to speak to people, to anyone, anywhere. Discovering how to shape a story. You want to write fiction, yup, but this must come first. This is your training. This is you, living and learning, until you have something worth saying to the world.

You get a rookie reporter job on terrible pay. But you stick at it. You learn your craft. You read every newspapers, every day. You learn shorthand, you pass the exams you need.

Journalism is a joy. It becomes your passion. Giving a voice to the voiceless. Representing the underdog.

You dare to believe, even bigger.

You start to cross over with camera crews and broadcast journalists, and you are intrigued by their work. So, watch every TV news bulletin, every day.

And when you see an advert, you apply to the BBC.

"Is there a better,
more balanced way?"

Photo by Bekir Donmez on Unsplash.com

Yes, they say. *We like you. Have a job, locally.* Go on screen. Go Live. Have an earpiece. A script. An autocue. A career. A big one.

You lean in.

You'll never make it onto the national news team, says Doubty. That's a bubble as big as a hot air balloon. Maybe, you agree. But it's worth a shot.

There are panel interviews, reporter scenarios, practical tests. Yes, they say, *we want you.*

Oh boy, you're really on your way now. You interview politicians, ministers ... even the Prime Minister! You work on election nights, on outdoor broadcasts, on special events. You stand in rain, snow, floods and heatwaves. You cover royal weddings, the world cup, the Olympics, Brexit.

But babies have come along. Beautiful and bamboozling, in equal measure. You're tired and you're torn. You want to be the best Mum, the best worker, and end up feeling you're doing nothing properly. For a while, you hit rock bottom. Doubty Gremlin grins as he stretched out a gnarly fingernail and …

P o p.

Is there a better, more balanced way?

You go part time, and ask to return to the local team. They don't want part timers. *I'll make it work*, you say. And you become the first ever part time woman to produce the flagship regional news programme. You blazed a trail, where others can follow.

Then you think, *I'm done.*

I did everything I wanted to, on screen and behind screen.

Now, to get back to my true love – writing books.

Doubty says – *Nah, you'll never make it.* The odds are against you.

Hardly anyone gets an agent, fewer still get into print. It's a pipe dream. The bubbliest of bubbles.

But, you're trying. You've got previous with this trying lark. Just you see. Doubty is always there, but you flick him away. One day you might even grind him under your foot until he's dust and – *voiceless*.

Because, you can do anything. You're you. A youey you, blowing your bubbles – up, up, up. And nobody else can blow bubbles like you.

Chrissy Sturt

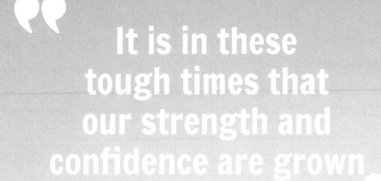

It is in these tough times that our strength and confidence are grown

Photo by Linus Nyland on Unsplash.com

HI YOU,

You don't know me, but I wrote this letter to you because I'm that someone who is proudly holding up a mirror to yourself, reflecting back all of the goodness, strength and kindness that you are.

I know it feels tough right now, like nothing is going your way and you just can't catch a break - it's OK. It's OK that you feel this way.

I'm here to remind you that whatever struggle it is that you're facing right now - you'll handle it. You always do. Trust yourself.

It is in these tough times that our strength and confidence are grown. They become the foundational and pivotal moments in this long, beautiful and unpredictable journey we call life. Ride the wave.

I just wanted to remind you of a few things from a few famous people that have walked a life and have turned out OK. They're not superhumans – they are just people, like you and me, but how they got to where they are is they didn't give in - they trusted the process and blossomed. Let's learn a thing or two from them together:

- Other people's opinion of you does not have to become your reality - Les Brown

- Never dull your shine for anybody else - Tyra Banks

- Big shots are only little shots who keep shooting - Christopher Morley

- Always be a first-rate version of yourself and not a second-rate version of someone else - Judy Garland

"I believe in you," whispered the reflection in the mirror <3

You have got this.

Diwa Sharma x

OPTIMISTIC FUTURES

DEAR LITTLE ME & FUTURE ME,

Trust that everything works out just as it's supposed to. Sometimes life might feel like too much, but I promise it all gets better.

Love and respect yourself, work hard, be vulnerable, above all, be kind. Don't let the negativity from others affect your kindness, they're just a little lost themselves. In life, people will come and go, don't let anyone treat you poorly, and always remember your worth. Caring about what others think of you is pointless. Most people don't even really know what they think of themselves - their opinions aren't your problems.

To have a small circle that you fully trust is all you'll ever need; as you get older, you will grow more grateful for the friendship found in your husband, your siblings, your parents. Family is forever, so care a little less about trying to prove yourself to those that aren't guaranteed to be there in the years to come. Value the ones that help to relieve the anxiety, not add to it, the ones who give you love without effort, and don't be afraid to tell them just how much you love them back, for tomorrow is not a guarantee.

The heartache, the silly boys and girls, it's all part of the learning curve. One day you'll find the one that matters most, the one that will understand you, grow with you, and love you for you. Never settle for anything less. Don't give up hope that you'll find the one that you'll never want to let go of and that will never let go of you. You deserve people who will love you just as much as you love them.

"Don't be afraid to come out of your comfort zone because that's where you'll thrive and make the very most out of life. Nothing good ever came out of staying in line - be different. Don't be afraid to fail, and don't expect to be a success overnight.

Never let anyone crush your dreams or tell you they're ridiculous, trust your gut and go for it because you'll always regret it if you don't. Life has no limits except for the limits we set ourselves.

Get a little lost, pack up, go explore the world, travel far away, learn about new cultures and make those memories that will last a lifetime. To travel will be the best money you will ever spend, for it will nourish your soul with wonder, growth and wisdom. You're allowed to be yourself, even if no one understands – it only has to make sense to you.

Lastly, love yourself fiercely. Learn to be your own biggest supporter and best friend but also remember you're never really alone. Have patience as everything will soon fall into place. Don't be so hard on yourself for feeling a little lost. Life would be so dull if you'd done it all already. You still have so much ahead of you. You just don't know it yet.

Love,

KeiKei Clothier (KeiKei Travels)

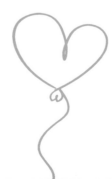

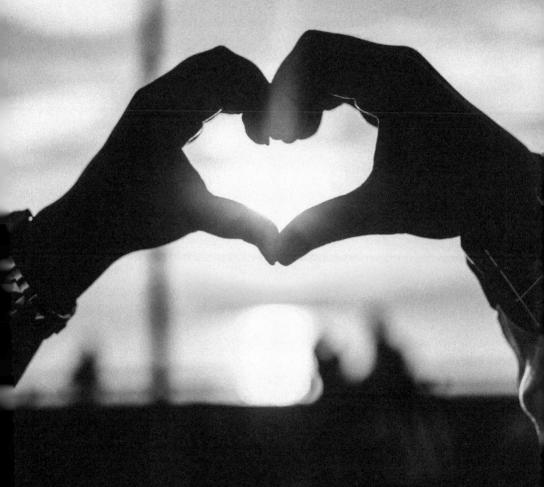

 Love yourself
FIERCELY

Photo by Tyler Nix on Unsplash.com

TO ANYONE BATTLING AN EATING DISORDER –

When I was told I had Anorexia Nervosa back in October 2019, I never thought it would happen to me.

I feel so lucky to be one of the survivors knowing how quickly life can be snatched away from you. There is no question that letting go of an eating disorder is one of the hardest things a person can do. It can feel like you are losing part of your identity, but through all the tears, sleepless nights, the thoughts of relapse, I continue to fight because recovery will give me my life back.

If I've learnt anything over the past few years, it's to always fight through whatever the world may throw your way. There's so much more to life than food, calories and exercise. I am slowly learning what it's like to be human again. What it means to make mistakes but this time not worrying too much and, most importantly, learning from them. I am learning how to just be in the moment, how to exist, how to understand that I cannot control life and life cannot control me. That I can only experience life in both its light and dark stages. I am learning how to laugh and cry and feel all the emotions that I haven't felt for so long. I am learning to accept me and simply believing in the person I am becoming.

My whole life, I have never been able to cry or show and feel emotion. For it was far too scary to do either, and I didn't know how to. Clinging onto my eating disorder felt so much safer. Anorexia was always there for me, a best friend. She never let me down.

It feels like I've lived several lifetimes worth of pain. And I'd become so deeply accustomed to it, I figured I'd live out the rest of my life as a shell of what I could've been.

I thought I'd always be broken. Someone who didn't know who they really were. Someone undeserving of life or help. But I have learnt that I am deserving and that I will find me eventually. I have learnt to believe in myself. I now see that I am not broken or damaged. That I am worthy of love, kindness and support.

I have been taught so many lessons, which I will forever keep close.

Lessons like: it's bravery, not perfection. It's self-compassion, not self-discipline. It's vulnerability that makes us stronger. It's finding the mid-ground that helps me to continue to move and grow.

I have been taught that I have the ability to change and the resilience to start again as many times as I need to and that everything doesn't have to be perfect or turn out the way I'd planned.

> Looking back, I understand now that I didn't need to be fixed or reassembled. I wasn't broken; I wasn't a mistake. All I really needed was to be seen and listened to.

For the first time in years, I can feel my mindset shifting from being in the clutches of Anorexia. I've gone from saying "I can't" to "What's the worst that can happen?" "It's too hard" to "I want a challenge." "I'm not ready yet, I need more time" to "There's no better time than now because the right time will never come."

You can start recovery whenever you want. You can start today, or next month or next year. But how much life will you lose in the time you wait for it to be the right time. There is never a right time or place to start recovery! No, you don't have to be sicker. You are already sick enough! You don't have to be underweight or have been an inpatient. You can start recovering even if you don't feel ready because let me tell you, it never feels right! The truth is you can change your life whenever you want. You can do something this week that will change your life forever. Don't be afraid to dive into recovery, as it's the only way you will ever get your life back! You never know what might just happen if you beat those demons forever.

People ask me, "How do you recover?" It's really hard to recover, I'm not going to sugarcoat that. You have lived with this illness for so long that you don't know anything else. How can you get your family and friends to understand when you don't even understand it yourself? I think to get better you really have to realize what you want in your life. What you want to achieve in the future as you cannot achieve this with an eating disorder. It really isn't possible, so you really truly do need to decide whether you want to live your life by an illness that one day will kill you, or do you want a better life and do things that you want to do and achieve whatever you want to do?

I couldn't be where I am today if I hadn't chosen recovery. I'm at university studying nutrition and psychology so that in the future I can help others just like me. I can't explain it, but recovery is the best thing you will ever do! I've got my life back, and I've learnt so much about myself over the past year, and you will do too! Please don't ever give up. Living is better than just surviving.

This letter is dedicated to everyone battling an eating disorder and those who sadly lost their fight to this deadly disease.

Thank you to the amazing NHS Lancashire and South Cumbria Eating Disorder Service, my family, my friends and my dog, Pippa, who have not only saved my life, but given me my life back.

Emily Pegg

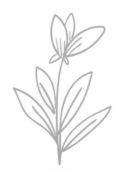

> **You can start recovery whenever you want. You can start today, or next month or next year. But how much life will you lose in the time you wait** FOR IT TO BE THE RIGHT TIME

DEAREST YOU,

We can think, plan, organize, wish, hope + pray for things to go a certain way, but they will always align how they need to for the highest growth.

Life is an ever unfolding of truth.

A deeper understanding of love.

A clawing back of the debris we accumulated along the way.

Revealing a more pure + raw heart. A dark space of vulnerability + pain — we are only ever looking to be more held, more heard, more felt.

I am learning compassion in the people I love + live alongside. I am seeing ways to become more compassionate through my life experiences. I am beginning to see that to be compassionate means to be truthful, raw + kind in every sense. To not shy away from it but to continually expand into its depths.

Compassion is something I have struggled to fully appreciate, acknowledge or receive. Yet its potency is profound + totally dismantling.

I apologize to anyone I ever caused pain to along the way. Please know, it is because I am healing too.

Anonymous Yoga Teacher

"Life is an ever unfolding of truth "

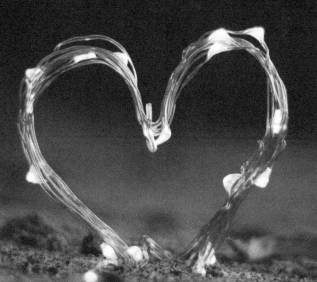

DEAR FRIEND,

I suppose I'm an old romantic at heart. Even though I should know better, I still adhere to the old school notion of true love. I tried deeply to dismiss it – telling myself it was all too complicated and that I couldn't possibly put my body through the angst of uncertainty that comes with it. It didn't work. When I was a child, I was often asked by teachers what I wanted to be when I grew up. Other children would excitedly say that they wanted to be firemen, princesses or police officers. I'd say that I wanted to be loved. I wanted the kind of love that my parents shared. The old-fashioned kind. The kind that doesn't exist much anymore. The kind that the fast-paced, ever-changing society that we live in today has deemed unnecessary.

A day out at the cinema watching *Moulin Rouge* when I was about ten years old cemented the timely nostalgia I so desired but hadn't yet realized. My best friend and I snuck into the movie screening after paying for a ticket to see *Shrek*, and boy were we in for a surprise. The historic grandeur of the costumes and the modern, over the top iteration of campy music was enough to have this little gay boy jumping for joy. I felt like I was being included in a mainstream love story for the first time.

> I was part of the generation of young city-dwelling gays that aspired to be part of the fab four Sex and the City girls, navigating our ways through the complexities of modern love in the big city. I fangirled out, dancing to the boogie of the salsa-flavored theme tune well into young adulthood.

From early on, I always knew that I'd been dealt a harsher hand at life. My mum confirmed this when I came out to her, and she wept. Not because I was gay, but because she knew I'd have a much harder time with it.

For a time, I set myself up believing the problematic notion that I'd never been truly happy because society didn't accept me. It was the mid-2000s, and I was deeply confused and dissatisfied with the status quo that was blankly staring me in the face. I was only sixteen, but I had a big fat grudge on my shoulders that I somehow needed to curb.

I had a plan, a concrete plan that couldn't go wrong – something only my own stupidity could have conjured up. I decided to be straight. Of course, I knew that deep down that I was a gay man, a proud one even. But the constructs of society were too much to challenge at a time when I felt like my ego was conquered. I wanted to fool the world into thinking that I was a straight man, get married, have two children and a semi with a white picket fence and a mortgage. Obviously, it didn't work out.

I didn't want to carry the weight of the world on my shoulders and come across as bitter, but I wanted to be afforded the same rights of passage that everyone else had. I grew up in a generation of nineties kids that were sold the idea of love through outdated and often problematic narrative arcs. I was extremely confused and hadn't even begun to experience love yet, but I was scared sh*tless nonetheless. It led me down a rabbit hole that I wish I could have protected myself from. I got into a string of bad relationships. One after the other and each worse than the last. It was like I was addicted to the low self-esteem I garnered from a life of bad decisions. I was intentionally letting myself be held back by the dangerous insecurities that I'd learned from childhood.

Something had to change, and then it clicked. Why didn't I think about this before? I mean, it's pretty simple, right? Love yourself.

To love others, you first need to love yourself. So that was my message for a little while. I'd go on a self-proclaimed journey of discovery and learn how to fall in love with myself.

I kept thinking, "What would Carrie Bradshaw do?" And then it was suddenly clear – I quickly realized that I was doing it again. I was projecting a Hollywood fantasy onto myself and feeling every bit accountable when it didn't go my way. My life was playing out like a Shakespearean tragedy and not even one of the good ones.

For the first time, I realized that not everything in my life would play out like a storybook. I learned that life was full of rough edges that couldn't be edited out in the studios of Los Angeles. The foggy lens of reality suddenly became crystal clear. There would be no more sugar-coated reality or fake facades for me. It's a moment that I think we all go through in one way or another. It was an eye-opener, to say the least.

With my newfound knowledge, I moved full throttle into the next phase of my life. I put my grudges behind me, unlearned most of my bad habits and focused on myself. I achieved a lifelong ambition and joined the Civil Service. I was working towards a career in estates management, and I was having the time of my life.

I was in a calm space mentally, had a good job and a goal that I was working towards. I had wonderful friends and a supportive family; I was finally on the up. No more was I bogged down by the fantasies I tried so hard to live up to as a kid. I had my imperfect life, and it was perfect. At no point was I looking for a man to come in and sweep me off my feet like Prince Charming, but that's exactly what happened.

Love means something totally different in modern times. It's no longer about the roles we were given to fulfil in the 50s, the American dream of three kids and a semi. It's no longer about making it work for the kids or worrying about what your friends will think. It's about being happy, and that's going to be different for everyone.

I can't say it enough, but we owe ourselves the fundamental human right of happiness wherever we find it. If you love your garden and it brings you happiness, who's to say that isn't as legitimate as a relationship. Our relationship with the world is what matters and whatever happens in-between is a bonus.

I can truly say that I am the happiest I have ever been. Not because I've found a life partner, and we now share a sense of solidarity, trust, faith and comradery; it's because we love the world that we live in individually and come together as a united unit as an expression of that love.

With so much love,

Anonymous

TO ANYONE WHO NEEDS TO REMEMBER TO NEVER GIVE UP –

On a Saturday afternoon in April 2005, I was taking part in something I loved; never did I dream it would end in disaster. Approaching 40 minutes into the game, I was on the receiving end of a late and high tackle. Instantly I knew, and so did the crowd, that I was in trouble.

I don't remember too much after that until I was being transported into an ambulance and heading for Hospital. It wasn't good, and the X-ray confirmed a double break of the tibia and fibula to my right leg. I was operated on and inserted through the bone was an Intramedullary (IM) rod from my knee to my ankle, where it remains today.

After months of rehabilitation, the hardest thing was not being told that I would never play football again or be able to run again. The hardest thing was learning to walk again, something that most people just take for granted every day. Getting the strength back and having the courage to take one step in front of the other and not fall over was so difficult, frustrating, and painful. I will never forget the day I took my first steps unaided. They may have only been five steps, but I burst into tears and broke down. As I said to myself, "I've done it," I only looked forward from that point.

I was back walking in four months unaided, I was told six months, and my next goal was to prove the doctors wrong and get back running. I did achieve that goal, but it took some time. I did it stages, treadmill and then soft grass, but I got back to doing a few kilometers. I was never going to get back up to marathon distances, but I was also never going to just accept that I couldn't run again.

Mind, power and determination will help you in difficult situations.

Paul Crang

113

TO ANYONE WHO STRUGGLES TO SEE A FUTURE – PLEASE DO NOT LOSE HOPE.

My earliest memory is having a panic attack. Don't get me wrong, I have some amazing childhood recollections too (such as dancing around my parent's living room in a sparkly gold leotard singing Abba songs – although come to think of it, that could have been any time in the last 42 years), but this is most certainly the first. I was five years old when my teacher asked me to stand up in assembly, telling the other children to look after me because my grandmother had just died. I can still feel the rush of adrenalin as I stumbled apprehensively to my feet, curious eyes piercing me from every angle. At that age, I had no way of articulating the sheer terror pulsing through my veins, but I instinctively knew I was in danger and had to escape. As I ran from the school hall sobbing in distress, little did I know that this was just the start of my battle with anxiety.

Throughout my childhood, a clear pattern emerged: any situation outside of my comfort zone would trigger panic attacks. The impact of this increased as I grew older, with simple activities like meeting new people or spending a night away from home causing me weeks of debilitating angst. I worked hard to hide my mental health issues from everyone, believing I was abnormal and that others would judge me if I confessed how broken I was. In secret, I sought various types of counselling, but nothing helped. I hated being me.

Then, with a stroke of incredible luck, I was assigned to an NHS psychologist who somehow, extraordinarily, helped me reframe everything I was experiencing. She supported me in understanding that it was ok and even normal to have these emotions, and we focused instead on coping mechanisms that would allow me to live the life I yearned for. In a handful of sessions, she helped me find a whole new path, one that has led me to where I am today. Self-acceptance is key, as is recognizing how many other people around us are suffering too. We are never alone.

I would be lying if I said I no longer experience anxiety, and I still have panic attacks even now. However, it no longer controls my life – I have travelled around the world, successfully delivered training to groups of strangers and even presented at a national conference in front of over 100 people. I show myself compassion and give myself permission to feel scared but find ways through that fear. Being open and talking about my problems is empowering – it never fails to amaze me how many people have had similar experiences. I write almost constantly, committing to paper the adrenalin that can sometimes threaten to swamp me. Some of these outpourings remain for my eyes only; some I share via a book blog under the pseudonym Bookaholic Bex. Most of all, I try hard to be my own friend – I would never have judged others as harshly as I judged myself, so it was time to give myself a break.

> Anxiety no longer defines me. It isn't an abnormality to be hidden away, but something that has made me a more empathetic, compassionate human being - and that is something I can truly be proud of.

And in my experience, the best people in my life are those who have been on a similar journey – mental health challenges are a superpower, not a disability. Now I have a future.

(It's just a shame that the sparkly gold leotard no longer fits).

Bookaholic Bex

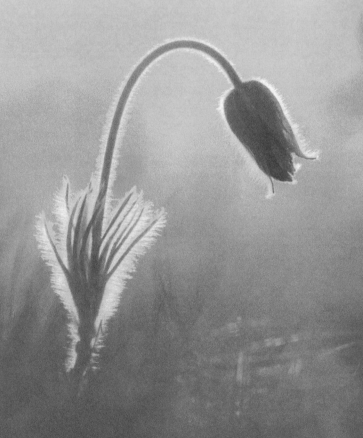

DEAR LAURA,

Nobody tells you what this is going to be like. When your whole world has come crashing down and all that's left is your delicate heart. Splintering more and more with each damned pulse.

You never realize how much you love someone until you are told you're going to lose them. Not "maybe," just a straight "you will lose this person" – there's nothing you can do. And your heart shatters. Because all those awful stories you hear about the beautiful family with the young daughter who's dying – they are the stories people use to tell your tale now.

> You learn how to pretend to be okay, and how to try and distract your mind for a while, but you never accept it. Maybe it's because your brain just can't comprehend losing the person who means the most to you in the world.

The day we found out, my heart just stopped. I was waiting for the punchline. Nobody really goes to the hospital and finds out they're dying. Do they? Looking back, I think my naivety was the only reason I didn't just collapse to the ground there and then.

The day of your surgery, you were so sick. I would have done anything to take your pain away from you and put it onto me, drained of feeling, so goddamn helpless all the time.

I remember waiting for the ambulance to come, stood outside in the rain at 5am holding a torch and screaming to the ground and God and Allah and Buddha and anyone who was listening to please not take you. I'm not religious, but someone clearly listened.

Seven days later, we were in a side room of a hospital ward being told there was nothing they could do.

The doctor's shirt was inside out, and you told him, right after the elusive glass ceiling had shattered over us all. I remember thinking how much that mundane comment helped me at the time, the one thing that stopped me curling up in a ball and never moving again.

You were dealing with it, so why shouldn't we?

Days after that merge into months of experimental drugs and treatment and 4am wake ups. Christmas trees in waiting rooms and hospital canteen food. Hurdles thrown from all directions.

Blurry morning voices and adrenaline-flooded veins were the sentimental feelings of that Christmas. The constant terror of trying to find an alarm clock ringing somewhere in a black, black room, a ticking time bomb ready to explode at any minute.

Then, clarity. Crystal clear days of laughter and sunsets and sunrise, nights under the stars in a hot tub with the three people I love the most in the world. Fresh linen sheets and telling stories lying next to you, warm baths while you watch TV on the bed behind me. Giggly stories and the kind of laughter that makes your stomach hurt for days afterwards.

David Attenborough and a gentle coal fire with a full tummy. Clear scans and happy car rides. Walks where we not only acknowledge the elephant in the room, but he's walking side by side with us, not scared anymore, just peaceful.

> Some days can still have that not-black-but-grey afterglow, and the feelings of battling against the tide to keep your head above water have only subsided a little. This unit is an iron strong one, and that isn't budging anytime soon.

My heart still spends most of the time in my mouth when we sit in waiting rooms or get tormented with yet another hurdle, but there's always you, little miss force-to-be-reckoned-with, facing everything thrown at us with a daring sense of positivity and a mindset ready to defy all odds.

This trip around the sun is the one we've dreaded most. The one we thought would bring nothing but heartache and numbness and black, black days. But here we all are, a little bruised but all still fighting. And that won't ever change.

Laura Mae, you are the bravest person I know. This year has put you through hell, yet you have dealt with it admirably. I am so, so proud to call you my sister.

Here's to next year being everything you want it to be and more, you deserve it. Happy 20th, Sis.

All my love, Gracie xxx

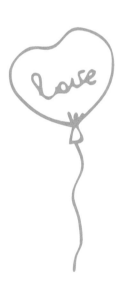

DEAR WENDY,

You weren't the brightest tool in the box, were you? I can totally appreciate you not enjoying school and not being able to wait to leave.

What was Dad thinking?

How were you ever going to "get" math and mental arithmetic with his bizarre methods of teaching?

Do you remember crying into your math book as he wheeled that stick at you? The ink spreading across the page with each tear drop?

Of course, that would make him even more annoyed and down that stick would come on your eight-year-old knuckles!

"You are fat, lazy and stupid! What are you?"

"Fat, lazy and stupid, Daddy!"

Having to repeat that mantra on almost a daily basis couldn't have helped your confidence in any subject, could it?

So, at senior school, you'd take any opportunity to skive off school, especially on the days you had double math!

Then, remember that afternoon when Mr. Brookes gave you detention to catch up with all your math missed?

Him standing behind you, saying, "Come on Wendy! This is easy!" and me replying, "I'm fat, lazy and stupid!" and then flinching, my hands protecting my head.

After school, you avoided any job that was going to entail any kind of math! Your best friend went to work at a local bank, and you couldn't imagine the horror of having to deal with all those figures!

You worked as a nanny with children of varying families. I think that was when you were at your happiest – with children.

Then you met John at the home of one of the families where you were a nanny.

You fell in love and went to work for John in his busy office.

He casually placed an adding machine in front of you to conduct the end of month figures and you had to run to the bathroom!

He tried to teach you, but you ended up a quivering wreck and that was the end of your time working in an office – forever!

You married and had three beautiful children.

You were wise not to pass your fear of numbers and hatred of math on to them.

Michael especially excelled at math and loved to help his sisters with their homework!

Listening to him teach the girls their times tables, you learned them, too.

You'd recite them by rote, and eight time seven was always fifty-six, as it was the one you never remembered!

By the time the children were school age, John had left, so, you decided to work with children again and became a child-minder.

Remember how you worried about sending invoices and calculating your hours worked with fees owed?

Ha-ha – you probably lost so much money through your calculating errors!

Twenty years later, the children having flown the nest, you wanted to give back to the children who you had helped rear.

> Poor mental illness in children had become a national threat. Children were becoming anxious, depressed, and suicidal.

You so wanted to help, but the thought of making a product for these children and setting up your own business frightened you!

Images of that dreaded adding machine and invoices!

You were so reticent about starting a course in business studies. How were you ever going to succeed being fat, lazy and stupid?

Supposing there were percentages?

But the thought of sitting back and doing nothing was even worse than the thought of having to deal with the above. You had a product in mind that could help children with their emotional wellbeing and mental health, and you wanted to get it out there!

You ought to have been a lot prouder of yourself than you were!

You stuck to that course and with the help of Michael, then in his twenties, learned about percentages, VAT, profit and loss, bookkeeping, statistics, mark-ups, markdowns!

Numbers were actually quite straightforward. Each calculation had a rule and sticking to that rule gave the correct answer every time!

It was fascinating! You loved it! You loved math!

You started your business in 2018, selling wellbeing resources and books to schools that helped children's emotional wellbeing and mental health.

The confidence you gained from completing the business studies course gave you the confidence to sell at the right price and still have a big enough margin! You knew what a margin was!

Three years on, today, do you still feel fat, lazy and stupid?

No. I didn't think you did.

You did good, Wendy!

Love,

Wendy

"
Numbers were actually quite straightforward
"

$-62\% + -42\% = \heartsuit$

$-73\% + -44\% = \ddot{\smile}$

A RIB CAGE IS NOT LOVE
By Daisy Moody

A hip bone is not validity.

A rib cage is not love.

My body is my armor,

and my skin a silken glove.

There is power in my stride

now I let myself be free.

My future is much brighter

now I let myself be me.

My features don't dictate

what type of person I can be.

My diamond heart that beats inside

means more than can be seen.

"Look at all your ugly flaws,"

said the Mirror on the wall.

Now I smile and say,

"I am the fairest of them all."

I accept that who I am cannot be

changed so easily.

I accept that I don't need to change,

I am who I should be.

My days are full of happiness,

since my mind is now at ease.

My thoughts are so much kinder,

'cause I finally love to eat!

A pizza is not ugliness.

A burger is not hate.

The more I live my life with joy,

the more I'm glad I ate.

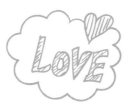

The Mists of Time

Long Ago

From:

Future Keith

A Place of Hope

Also Leeds

DEAR PAST KEITH

How's it going? Actually, forget I asked. I already know.

I am aware that, in receiving this letter, you may be hoping for some specific advice on upcoming events. What to do, what not to do, and *ahem* who to do it with given half the chance. Sadly, as you and I both know, the rules of time travel would render such advice worthless after the first event. The ripples of cause and effect would change the future enough that nothing else would happen in the same way, and you would instead be left with a big list of what might have been, much like I have in my head right now.

Instead, I would like to offer you some guidelines that have proven useful to me over the years. Some are borrowed, some are my own, but all have been shown to have a grain of truth in them. May they help guide you into making good and beneficial choices, whatever they may be.

(Presented in no particular order)

1. When someone shows you who they are, believe them.

2. The hardest part of ending any relationship is letting go of who you thought that person might one day be.

3. Don't worry about what other people think of you, because chances are they seldom do.

4. Don't accept criticism from someone you wouldn't go to for advice. (This will become especially relevant when internet "trolls" become a thing.)

5. Don't self-reject. Be it a date, a job, or a competition, it's up to them to say no. Also, don't fear the no's. They often hurt less than you imagine, and the pain never, ever lasts.

6. It's easier to ask forgiveness than permission.

7. Save your money. At least 10% every month. I'll thank you later.

8. Likewise, don't smoke, don't drink, eat well, and get some exercise. You only get one body, and you need to take care of it.

9. Don't waste your time trying to make other people happy. Their happiness is fleeting, and you'll only make yourself miserable in the long run.

10. It's much better to have a party and invite other people than it is to try and wangle an invite to someone else's. You can take this both literally and as a metaphor.

11. There are no difficult decisions. You know what needs to be done. The only time we get into trouble is when we don't like the conclusions we have come to.

12. Never argue with an idiot, they'll drag you down to their level and then beat you with experience. Also,

13. Never take an idiot on a long journey. You'll always find one along the way.

14. Don't hug people you want to be intimate with. Hugs are for friends and family. Stick with a kiss on the cheek, for now.

15. Tradition is peer pressure from dead people.

16. The three worst reasons to do anything are loyalty, tradition, and patriotism.

17. A wise man knows when to advance, when to retreat, and when to stand still. Sometimes doing nothing is the greatest skill of all.

18. Where you focus your energy is where you will see results. This applies to both the positive and the negative alike.

19. Anger and hate all come from a place of fear. Do not ignore them, but do not let them dominate your life.

20. Whatever happens, it's better to make choices than it is to just go along with everyone else. It's easier to live with your own mistakes than it is someone else's.

21. In a world where you can be anything, be kind, especially to yourself.

And there you have it. Not an exhaustive list, but plenty to be going on with for now. I'm sure, over time, you'll be able to add a few more of your own.

Best of luck, mate. It won't always be easy, but it will be interesting, and if you ever think things aren't going to work out remember: everything will be alright in the end, and if it's not alright, then it is not the end.

Cheers

Future Keith

PS. Okay, I said I wasn't going to do this, but here goes. In 1998, whilst working for the Edinburgh Film Festival, you're going to meet a Scots lass named Rosie. Ask her out as soon as you can, because by the time you work out how lovely she is she'll be seeing someone else, then the festival will be over, and you'll never seen her again.

I'm not saying she's the love of your life or anything – I've no idea. But you will always wonder, and there's nothing worse than an itch you can't scratch, so ...

Everything will be alright in the end, and if it's not alright, IT'S NOT THE END

LETTER TO MY 16-YEAR-OLD SELF –

You didn't think you would make it.
You don't think anything can change.
You thought your life had a fixed path.
A one-way street down misery lane.

You try and try, yet nothing feels enough.
You feel unlovable, unworthy, and that life is tough.
You are told to try harder, to never give up.
You feel weak and stupid that nothing adds up.

I am you from the future.
I came here to say.
You are worthy,
You are special, in every way.

You learn to accept yourself.
You find out who you are.
Accepting help becomes okay as you learn to
trust people more each day.

You can ground yourself when things are rocky.
You can rest and restore without shame.
You learn it's not your fault.
You can feel your feelings.
You can share your pain.

You feel heard and comforted without fear.

Growing without shame.

You grow stronger day by day.

Helping others feel the same.

You create a space to feel accepted, heard and understood.

You learn it's not your fault you did everything you could.

You prove to others hopes and dreams can come true.

You are starting to believe in the power of YOU.

A bright beam of sunshine.

A kind voice to hear.

A dose of kindness and compassion.

A friend who many hold dear.

Your experiences were painful.

This is true.

Yet, they created the woman in front of you.

Hold on. It is worth it. It is better. It does change.

Many Thanks

Nikky Reed, founder of #NOLABELS

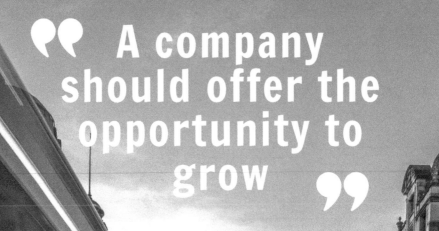

A company should offer the opportunity to grow

DEAR EARLY-IN-CAREER PROFESSIONAL:

As a father, as a mentor, as a CEO of a global shipping and mailing company, I have seen firsthand the challenges young people face when starting out in business. It's definitely a new world from when I was just starting out.

When I started working decades ago, I was at a company with a promise of a job for life.

> As a CEO today, I can't guarantee our people a job forever, but I can promise them that I will provide the opportunities to continue to evolve their skills. That's a value proposition for today.

When you are looking to join a company, understand what their promise is. What they value. Will you be given the opportunity to continue to evolve your skills? Because if you think about how quickly the marketplace is changing and how much change you're likely to encounter during your working years, it's going to be wild. The skills that you have today will not be the skills that you need in five years or ten years. To have a vital career will take your commitment to learn and develop as well as the support from your leaders to try and do interesting projects and expand your skillset.

At Pitney Bowes, we are a company that not only says we care about learning and development, but we actually mean it. We have a program called EIC program. It's an early-in-career program that gives new career professionals an opportunity to work in a global cohort on real-world business issues. Also, talent discussions are consistent and constant here as we want people to have a path forward.

While no company today can promise a job for life, what a company should offer is the opportunity to grow as you move along your career path and your future.

Choose wisely, and good luck in your career.

Marc Lautenbach, CEO, Pitney Bowes Inc

FOR MY NEPHEW,

My lovely nephew, who is kind at his core
Someone who makes you laugh - that's for sure
If you don't know him, don't be nervous, he can be quick-witted from the fore.

I have witnessed you develop into a sound, talented young man
A real friend to many, a star when it matters, I'm a true fan
Like any teenager, he can be annoying... like an unwanted orange tan.

It gives me great pleasure to call you my nephew
I like it when we spend time together, talking about stuff and deciding what's on the menu
You are truly loved, the distance to the moon & stars... I must tell you.

You brighten up my life, that's for sure

Being 16, I wish you sweetness in your life, for you to adore
In all that you do and in what you will become, but please no strife or chords that don't chime.

I look forward to the day you will eat more vegetables
And to hear about your adventures
About the things you have learnt, what makes you happy & brightens up your day.

But please be assured, I'll take the whole person as you are
Someone who means the world to me
Which incidentally is never in any doubt.

Love, your auntie x

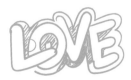

A LETTER TO A BRAVE READER –

To the person who is reading this…

You are going to be the best at life, defeat it, conquer it, achieve it.

Fearless and brave, that's what you are.

You are ambitious, a fighter, courageous.

Whatever you put your mind to, you are capable of.

Your heart and soul are kind and delightful.

I know you don't know me, but I am here for you, I care for you.

Hope will find you.

I want you to know you are safe.

You are wanted.

You are unbelievably amazing.

You belong.

You light up this world.

You will and can overcome anything.

You have so much potential.

I'm so proud of you.

No matter what you are going through, you will be okay.

To the person who is reading this, you will be the best at life, defeat it, conquer it, achieve it.

Savannah Kealey

HEY, MY DEAR FRIEND!

I heard that you weren't feeling your usual self. I just wanted to send you this letter to let you know that it's okay to not always be in the most happy, secure place… we've all been there, let me assure you!! Wow. The past few years have been wild, right?!

Sometimes, life gives us these challenges and jagged changes to test our might, to test our willpower and to show us all the places where we can expand and grow beyond what we're currently settling for.

Wouldn't life be boring if we coasted, and everything was sweet and easy?

Surely you wouldn't know true happiness if you hadn't experienced sorrow. A soul sister once told me that there will always be two magpies… "one for sorrow, two for joy". And it's true! There can exist no sorrow without joy. Life constantly works in polarities. And maybe at this moment, you're feeling something "bad" because of the good that's coming!! The lower we go, the higher we fly. Trust and surrender to the ride.

It's totally okay to not feel 100%, 100% of the time. You're human! And a human has this intense layer called the emotional body. So many feelings, sensations, emotions. Arising and dissipating. Try not to cling. Try not to hold on to the heavy - maybe it's just coming up for you to let go, to release? Maybe there's a little part of you that just needed to be heard and felt so that it could be free, and you could move on with more understanding, more depth, more heart? Maybe this challenge is actually forging you a new path ahead?

I promise you that life will always bring you what you need, and times won't always be hard. It might feel like you've been stuck in it foreverrrrr, but being dramatic is for actors. Haha! Let me give you a task: find one thing each day to be grateful for. Just one! Do one thing that makes you feel really joyful or alive. And offer one nice act of service for someone else each day. If you can do that daily, those small acts will build momentum and soon, you'll be right out of that hole you've dug deep down into.

Sitting into the feelings and looking at our shadow is crucial work, for sure. But please know when it's time to release, to move on. Allow yourself to open your heart and eyes to the magic, to the beauty, the glory and the freedom of this incredibly magnificent life.

Stagnation is so easy to get stuck in, and it can feel like a lifetime to move on, but take each day as it comes and promise yourself that you'll do 1% better each day. Be kind to where you're at and trust that it's part of this incredibly confusing and magical experience that is life.

Don't cling to what you're going through. Embrace it, move it through you and transform yourself. There is always time, there is always hope, there is always enough. Life can change in an instant; why not make the future something worth fighting and working for?

Don't be hard on yourself though, mate – you're going through enough. Listen to your thoughts - what ways do you speak to yourself? Offer yourself compassion, always. Remember, no matter what, life is always working out for the better, and you can trust that. So, surrender to the path and focus on this moment, because now is all there really is.

You have massive power, you know? It's within your mind. When you look at something from a different angle, question it in a different way or bring curiosity in, what you're looking at will change. Your mind is more powerful than you believe right now. Life can, and will, be what you make it.

So, dream big and put that epic imagination to good use. Play whenever you can (who told us playtime was for kids?!) and bring back daily moments of joy. However small.

Start where you are. Use what you have. Do what you can.

Life is waiting with open arms for you, my dear friend!! Seize it and leave a blazing trail behind you. Because that's what we all came here for. To make history and bring our creations into reality. The Universe will support you – just make the first move!

Robyn Allan

To THE oNE WHO CAUSED ME PAIN –

I can feel my anxiety rising, I can see the terror in my eyes.

You abused me, over and over. You conditioned me to believe that toxic behavior is normal in relationships. That I deserved to be treated this way.

Instead of running a mile, I bonded with you. I desperately wanted to be loved by you. I was addicted to you.

You manipulated me – you hurt me, started to cry and said you were sorry. You were the perfect partner, doing the housework, buying me nice things. I believed you, every time.

As the bonding deepened, I unwittingly gave you more power, resulting in further manipulation and abuse.

It took me years to realize that I was in a toxic relationship and that you are a narcissist. Even then, I felt that I could not live without you, you were the love of my life.

But I am living without you. With the help of family, friends, and domestic violence organizations, I have broken the Trauma Bond.

It is not always easy, and I did not go easy on myself – you can see that by the scars on my arms. Sometimes, I am hyper-vigilant. I feel on edge when I am out shopping, at home watching TV. Loud noises startle me. I am distracted when I am assessing for potential threats.

However, I have a safety plan and a good support network to help me through these difficult times, and I am looking forward to my future. Because I deserve a better future.

Karen D

I am looking forward to my future. Because I deserve a better future

A LETTER TO MY 17-YEAR-OLD SELF –

You might not listen to this; sometimes, you don't like to take advice from people in their 40s. That's ok. People in their 40s don't always have good advice, and they don't always know best.

But on this occasion, I do know what I'm talking about because I *am* you – older, fatter and a bit wiser… calmer, kinder to myself and others, and with a slightly posher telephone voice. But I am you, and you are me, and I so wish I could have sat down with you and said this stuff at the time.

Firstly, you need to know that you can't be perfect, and more importantly, no one expects you to be. Whenever life feels hard, or you're uncertain what to do, you just need to behave in a way you can feel proud of when you look back. That is all we have.

There are worries that take up your headspace now, things that feel so huge and heavy they sit on your rib cage at 2am like a stone. I promise you that most of these things get smaller and lighter as you get older. It's hard to imagine now, but in a few years' time, you will not be worrying about your sexuality, or your exams, or your weight, or who might hurt you, or whether and where you belong.

I'll level with you, though: some stuff gets bigger over time. You will care more with every passing year about whether you are making the world a better place. It sounds cheesy, but it happens. It can be a pressure – make it a sense of purpose instead. You will worry more about other people; some days, it will be physically painful how much you care about someone else. Lean into it – it's because you love them, and that is a gift.

 Speaking of love… Don't let sex do the work of love. It is just not the right tool for the job.

You will not stop missing the people you've lost, but you will find a way to miss them without it destroying you. Some days you won't even think about them – don't feel guilty about this, it is what they want for you.

Let's talk about choices. You don't always make good ones; that's ok. You will learn to make better ones – and by this, I don't mean choices that other people always approve of, but you will increasingly make choices that make you feel happier, safer and healthier. Start now by asking yourself what advice you would give to your best friend or baby sister. If you can love yourself as much as you love them, you will give yourself better advice. You will still make some dodgy choices when you are older, sorry. But you will make them less often, and you will get better at repairing any damage, and you will come to understand that some of the "choices" you made when you were young were not actually choices – they were the best you could do in a bad situation. Forgive yourself.

> **Don't let any opportunity pass you by; failure is temporary, but regret sticks around.**

Oh, and you know That Family Member that occupies so much of your thoughts now? You haven't failed to build a relationship with them, so don't write it off just yet. You just need to come back to it at a time when you're both feeling braver, when you've both let the bruises heal. It might take a couple of attempts; hang in there.

However, I'm afraid there will be other relationships that still aren't resolved even by the time you're my age. You will find a way to make that ok too. You will learn to accept that some people can't be in your life because it is not good for you. And you will eventually understand that this is not a failure on their part or yours – it's just a rational decision, like avoiding foods that give you a rash.

You will meet some people in your life who will help you be your best self. Listen out for them; they aren't immediately obvious. They see something in you that you don't yet see yourself – like a flash of diamond in the rock-face. They will set you challenges that you think you can't do; you are wrong. They will ask you questions that are hard to answer; try anyway. They will sometimes be a bit tough on you; trust their motives. They will see past your carefully constructed facade and know that you are more scared and vulnerable than you appear. This will make you feel angry and scared; push through this – they will catch you if you fall.

Right now, it feels like you have no power or influence. It will creep up on you, just like grey hairs. When you notice that some people seem to listen to some of what you have to say, make sure you're saying something useful.

When you find your voice, speak up for those who can't. Always punch up.

And drink more water. Seriously. Your 40-odd-year-old self will be very grateful.

By anonymous

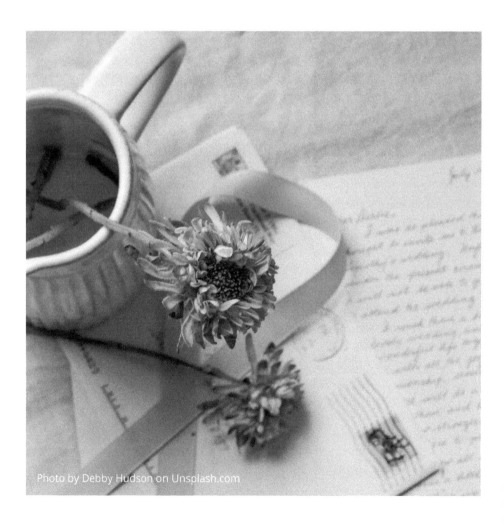

Photo by Debby Hudson on Unsplash.com

DEAR ME,

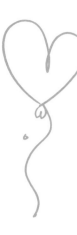

How are you doing? I know not many people ask

I know right now our world is a scary place

I know how broken you are and the tears you hide

I know you're struggling but still wearing a smile

I won't say our journey is going to be easy or short

I think we will have to fight for a while

But I wanted to remind you

That we have made it through bad chapters before

We have weathered the storm so many times

And each time we come back stronger, braver and

More wise

There will be a time when you don't hide tears in

Your eyes

There will be a time when you wear a real smile

And things are OK for a while ...

From,

Me

DEAR 16-YEAR-OLD ME,

I'm writing this from your future. I know it sounds unbelievable, not just the bending of the space/time continuum, but the possibility that there will be a future, that you'll make it. But you do – and it's glorious! Well, lots of it anyway. I'm not going to lie and pretend it's all great, because it's not. Unfortunately, life doesn't work like that. Forgive the cliché, but it's a rollercoaster with amazing highs and devastating lows. But you get through it all because you're so much stronger than you realize.

Right now, you're hitting hit rock bottom. I wish I could be back there with you at the hospital, holding your hand, letting you know that I see you, and I understand. A cry for help, that's what people call it. You hate the term. I still do.

It feels like life will never be bright again, but this fateful time triggers the start of a new beginning. The counsellors you are forced to see do help, not at first, as you are very good at pretending you're ok. But in the following years, you keep mulling over their advice and slowly but surely take it to heart and work out your own, more positive coping mechanisms. It's a journey, not a quick fix, but you need to have faith in yourself because you can do this. You will do this. By your early 20s, you've broken the cycle, and you don't look back.

You get a degree, travel the world, volunteer where you can, fall in love (lots!), find the one and get married (yes, I know you don't believe in marriage, but things change and trust me, he is wonderful!). You run two businesses. Most amazingly, you have two phenomenal children who blow you away every day with their imperfect perfectness. For them, you want to be the best person you can be. They are the ultimate proof the world is not better without you.

All of this might seem unattainable right now, but it's coming, I promise you. You just have to live it. If you only take one thing from this letter, it's this – please stop putting so much pressure on yourself to be perfect. It's ok not to be, as none of us are. To tell you the truth, it's something I'm still working on. But we'll get there.

Clare Giltrow

Please stop putting so much pressure on yourself to be perfect

DEAR YOUNG PERSON, FRIEND AND COMMUNITY MEMBER,

My name is Andi Brierley. I am a 40-year-old University Teacher at Leeds Trinity University. I am a husband to a wonderful Spanish wife and proud father of a 5-year-old daughter. I live what could only be described as quite a normal everyday life with little to no drama. Prior to becoming a University Teacher, which only happened very recently, I have spent 15 years working with children and young people involved in the youth justice system. In more recent years, specifically children in the care of the Local Authority involved in youth justice to inspire them to have better outcomes.

Not a particularly unusual story to start, you must be thinking. Well, my life certainly didn't start out in a way that ever made me believe that I would write that first paragraph. In fact, the reason I write this letter to you is to explain my unusual journey into my role and how you should never give up on yourself, just in the same way I didn't give up on myself.

My journey started out being born to a 17-year-old mother who had just left a children's home. My mother was abused and taken into care, but she never settled. At that time, in 1981, there was no legal requirement of the Local Authority to support those children leaving care which left mum vulnerable and alone. Mum wanted to love and to be loved as we all do and very quickly had my brothers and sisters, which meant she had five children at the age of 24.

As mum had been in care herself and constantly ran away, she didn't feel comfortable asking for support from services such as social care. This was mainly because she was worried that services would find out that she was not coping with being a mother to five children under the age of eight with no support. This meant mum would often take support from mainly men, but also females that were also finding life challenging for different reasons. People with mental health issues involved in crime and substance misuse were pretty much the only people that ever came into my home.

Mum also struggled to stay in one place, and if ever there was a violent incident, she developed debt, or she wanted to escape from a violent

> **Lack of connection with myself was fueling my loneliness** AND DISCONNECTION

partner, mum would move. By the age of seven, social care got involved due to suspected abuse and neglect. Over a period of seven months, it was evident that the level of adversity, abuse and neglect that we as children were experiencing was damaging, and we were taken into care and later separated, leaving me as the only child.

Mum did everything she could to get us back, and after 18 months, we returned home, and mum became very good at pretending to social care that things had improved. Eventually, they stopped the support, but things stayed the same. People that came into our home were always struggling with their own life challenges, and mum continued to move due to violence, a result of having such people around our family. By thirteen, I had lived in eighteen different family and foster homes. I had fallen so far behind my peers educationally (I won't say friends as although I spent time with other children, they were never very close for obvious reasons.). My behavior in school by the age of thirteen started to become challenging, and by fifteen, I was excluded. This was mainly because I started to take things from school for drugs.

I started smoking cigarettes by eleven and doing drugs by twelve, trying to manage what I can only describe as an internal pain. But, because I was only young, I didn't really understand why I was feeling so low in mood. This led to me becoming a drug addict after being expelled from school at the age of fifteen, which left me vulnerable. Adult drug dealers then took advantage of my vulnerability and convinced me to sell drugs for them. This was not difficult as I didn't have the supportive adult relationships to protect me from this. Because I was an addict by this point and needed to buy drugs, it seemed like something I could do that wouldn't directly hurt others. Of course, it wasn't long before I was arrested and sent to a Young Offender's Institution for two eighteen months sentences and while alone, I felt I deserved this because I was a bad person.

> I convinced myself that was I less deserving than other people and found myself in and out of prison and on and off drugs from the ages of seventeen to twenty-three.

While in prison, it was not interventions or programs that helped me. It might seem difficult to understand, but even in the darkest times, music helped me believe in myself. Many songs did this, but specifically, a song by Kelly Price called "Love Sets You Free" helped me remember that before I loved other people, and certainly before I allowed other people to love me, I first had to learn to love myself.

Throughout this journey of adversity, I had lost connection with myself. This lack of connection with myself was fueling my loneliness and disconnection with others that was driving my behavior and drug addiction. It is the lack of connection that makes a childhood traumatic, not the events. I always knew I was a good person. I know every child and young person is good at heart. Many of us, for different reasons, lose faith in ourselves and faith in others. When this happens, look for the hope around you. Hope comes in different ways for different people, but first, remember that you, like my mum, deserve to love and be loved, as do we all.

Andi Brierley

"Dark days don't last forever"

said Summer.

"Have you forgotten

that the seasons change?"

Anonymous

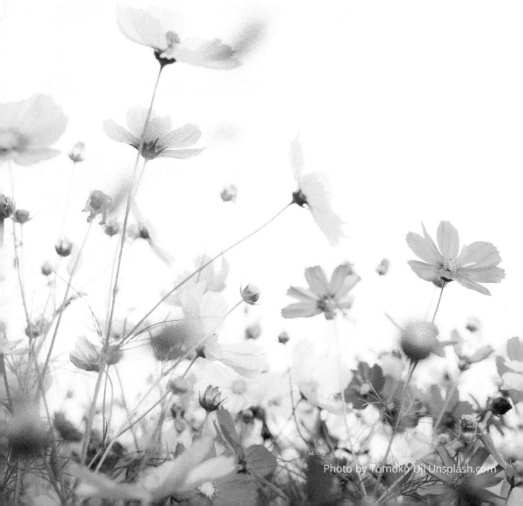

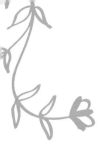

TO ANYONE WHO FEELS LIKE GIVING UP

Patience and not giving up are important life skills. Being patient and continuing to work hard at anything in life, no matter how tough it gets, will pay off in the long run; the key is to not give up in the process.

I always believe if you keep moving forward, step by step, no matter how hard things get, you will see how far you have come. For example, during my sporting journey in the early days, I had many setbacks and injuries due to me not being patient. I didn't learn to start off with and nearly gave up, but I did learn from my mistakes. When I look back at when I first started, I wasn't able to swim and kept getting injured. But, I kept going.

Now, when I look at what I have achieved – such as becoming a European Age Group champion – I realize how far I have come.

> So, you see, just keep moving forward, and give yourself credit for how far you've come.

Kind regards,

Yiannis Christodoulou

DEAR NEW FRIEND,

I would love to introduce you to my old friend. Fear not, they will not argue with you, and you don't need to dress up, or dress down – just be yourself. But before I do, let me say how we became friends.

For years, I struggled. I was diagnosed with complex PTSD, and my self-worth, confidence, and value were down in the dumps. No, they were down a black pit of despair. People said there is light at the end of the tunnel. I couldn't see the end – indeed, I was so far in I didn't even know where I entered.

I struggled with my trust in others, and I had given up on trusting myself. Altogether, I put myself in some stupid, risky, dodgy situations.

Then, when I failed to find ways to express myself in words, I discovered or rather rediscovered a friend who had always been nearby available to help, but whom for years I had ignored.

My friend, one I could trust no matter what, who never did anything I didn't permit, never answered back, never interrupted, never gave platitudes for answers, never went away. My friend required and wanted nothing from me except some attention and a battery. My friend, you see, was my camera. Okay, I confess I now have a number of friends, from the camera phone to slightly posher friends with complicated dials and interchangeable lenses.

> My camera and I have a trusting relationship born
> out of knowing each other and having a like desire
> to use the artist's canvas, the one before us each
> day, called Mother Nature.

My camera and I have become an "us." We are a team. Together, we step into the world with no expectations other than to allow the wonders of Mother Nature to show off her diversity and for us to do our bit and receive what she does as a gift of grace for that moment, that minute, hour or day.

Receiving what is before us as a gift, without judgement or apparent value of subject, just receiving with gratitude has transformed, uplifted, inspired and changed my life.

From darkness to light, despair to hope, dim tunnels to vibrant streets together, my camera and I have become the closest and most trusted of friends.

> I don't need fancy gear, just my phone and an open mind. I don't need to seek the images, just receive the ones each moment brings.

In such times, the mind opens, the fog lifts, the complex becomes clear, worries are seen for their reality, and my heart and mind are at peace. In such times you can almost photograph the sound of distant birds, photograph the aroma of fresh-cut grass. And for me, in the inner city, each corner, each shadow, each place of light, each touch of shade become places of questions and answers received to the silent photographer.

It is a relationship I treasure and one available to all. Yes, all ... just look at the thing called a phone, see the camera and discover a friend. You will never regret it, and if you are like me, you might just find it changes your life.

Ade Wyatt

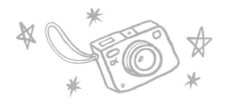

To WHOEVER NEEDS To SEE THIS,

I want to share something that I've learned. Something that can hopefully shine a little bit of light on a path that, right now, might seem shrouded in darkness. I want to talk about the impact of a conversation.

Sharing thoughts, feelings and ideas has enabled humanity to conquer the world. We did not evolve in isolation; even the most successful of our species needed some help and validation along the way. That's why I want to communicate exactly why I think conversations and connection matter so much, particularly when it comes to our ability to feel happy and healthy in life.

> The message on speaking up is out there - most of us now know that if we're struggling with a problem, we are supposed to talk about it if we want to feel better.

From personal experience, I know it isn't always that easy, though, for a variety of reasons. We might not wish to burden others with our issues. We might fear the way we will be perceived. It might have consequences for our ability to fit in, our education, our job prospects, or our family situation. We don't want the dreaded "snowflake" label. Or maybe we just simply don't have the words to explain what we're feeling yet. Speaking up and engaging in dialogue around how we feel can be challenging, confusing, awkward, embarrassing, upsetting or all of the above.

Whilst I acknowledge this reality, though, I cannot express enough how important it is that we keep trying to normalize these conversations.

Finding that outlet can change a life. It can even save a life.

When I think about the impact of certain conversations on my own lived experience of mental ill-health, I can say that talking to others has transformed what goes on in my head.

I first felt the onset of what I would later understand to be an anxiety disorder at a point in my late teens, only a year or so into my military

" Finding that outlet can change a life. It can even SAVE A LIFE **"**

career, when everything should have been going great. I was well-regarded in my workplace, received a swift promotion and was handed a high-profile position. After a few months, however, finding that the job wasn't really for me and feeling increasingly cut off from my friends and family, I noticed some physical symptoms of anxiety. I didn't understand what was happening for a while and thought that I might have some sort of mystery virus! Time spent concentrating on my churning stomach, pounding head, and frequent dizziness only made things worse, to the point where I would simply shut myself away from anything and everything, eyes closed, waiting for sleep.

After a few months of feeling like this and struggling in silence – I got incredibly lucky. A chance meeting with an amazing person (who now happens to be my wife) provided me with an outlet to share these concerns. Just being able to talk to somebody about how weird and panicky I would feel in certain situations was helping. It also gave me the confidence to be a little more open with the doctor, who, to that point, had received a carefully edited list of my symptoms due to my embarrassment and denial.

My up-and-down journey with my mental health has continued right up to the point at which I write this letter, but I am profoundly grateful for those early opportunities to open up and share what was going on with me. I have since experienced further spikes in anxiety and depressive episodes, usually based on an imbalance somewhere in my lifestyle, but I have always tried to remember how much lighter I feel just by talking to someone about what's going on.

I know how lucky I have been to have the support of friends, family and colleagues, to all of which I know I can open up if I feel the need.

Even if you don't think that you have that kind of support network in place, though, you can still access the healing power of a safe, non-judgmental conversation.

Services such as Samaritans are available 24/7, 365 days a year, to provide exactly that. Mind, the UK's national mental health charity, facilitate amazing peer support groups for those in need. Sometimes all we need to clear the fog is a listening ear to help us feel less alone and walk with us, to validate what we are feeling and show compassion. Thankfully, as we become more understanding around our mental health and wellbeing as a society, the future looks increasingly bright.

I want to finish this letter by offering some advice to those who might be worried about someone but feel unsure on how to start the conversation. My message to you is this – authenticity will always shine through. Language is important, but if your genuine desire is to help someone, that will prove far more powerful than the particular words you use. Simply letting that person know that you see them, you are there to listen and that you care about them is a potentially life-changing act. It is something that, if we all commit to it, can make the world a much nicer place to be.

Have the conversation.

Mike O' Hara

Founder of Start Within and RAF Veteran

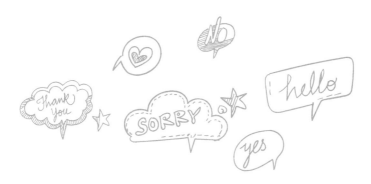

DEAR ALCOHOL,

I did not stop to think when friends asked me for a drink,

but then,

one drink led to ten, and to unwanted behavior,
the kind of which I do not savor.

Next morning, I look at my scars, realizing I have forgotten
quite how I got them.

Each day I cry,
I feel so low from living high.

But I won't let this wonderful life pass me by,
I know that it can end in the blink of an eye.

DEAR CLEAN LIVING,

You are so very giving.

I love you more every day,

and hope that you will stay.

Fantasies of how bad recovery could be,

nearly hampered it for me.

But I know that the pain is not permanent,

and I am determined,

to be fit, healthy and strong.

I want to enjoy life and live it long.

Karen Dillon

Get ready to fly – there are exciting times ahead

DEAR ME,

It'll be a shock to find a letter from your future self here, but I wanted to let you know that life doesn't always go according to plan and isn't always easy, but that deep inside you have the most amazing strength and ability to get through the challenges ahead and emerge happy and successful the other side.

Over the years I've learnt several things I wish I'd known when we were in our late teens and early twenties, but in case it helps I'll share them here.

> Regardless of what you might think, you ARE good enough. Don't compare yourself with others all the time.

It doesn't matter whether they seem physically more attractive, intellectually superior, or more successful because that's about them. You are you. And they may have all kinds of emotions and struggles in their life you know nothing about and be secretly wishing they are you!

Don't keep moving the goal posts. I know you only too well and as soon as you look as if you're going to succeed you set a new, more difficult target, so that you're set up to fail. Decide a goal. Write it down and give yourself a small reward if you get to it. Then you can set a new challenge. And those rewards don't need to be expensive or known about by anyone else. You'll find reading a book for ten minutes whilst you drink a cup of tea can be just what you need!

Be brave and take a chance. In your early 30s you were highly successful in your career after a meteoric rise through the ranks, you had (and still have) a brilliantly supportive husband. You had plenty of money. You were buying yourself expensive treats like diamond jewelry. But above all else, you were utterly miserable. Why? Because you'd lost sight of who you were. You were a wife, a dutiful daughter, a Head of Department, a supportive sister, a caring daughter-in-law and so many other personalities that actually you never had time to be you. It took physically paralyzing yourself briefly from overworking, being unable to move let alone work, for several weeks to make you realize public success, status and lots of money do not equate to happiness. You took a chance. You gave up your job, more than halving your household income and you managed. It was tough at times, but the result was a happier you – and, ironically a few years later, a much wealthier you too!

> **What you learnt at that time is that actually you are amazing.**

For example, you were working full time in a stressful job on the day your mother-in-law died, your dad was rushed into hospital with a suspected heart attack and your Mum passed out when you took her to visit him, and you could easily have crumbled. You didn't. You coped. And you keep on coping now.

Only now, you know it doesn't matter if you're not coping. It doesn't matter what people think of you as long as you know you've done your best, been kind to others and have been true to yourself. When the times get tough again, you now know you can ask for help. And you also know that it's OK to say no to someone when they ask you to do something you really don't feel up to doing.

Get ready to fly – there are some exciting times ahead!

Look after yourself.

Love

Me

Linda Hill

DEAR YOUNGER SUE,

It's 1996. You've sold your first short story to a national magazine. It took you three years, over thirty different submissions and a writing course, but your name's going to be in print and you have a cheque for £65. Congratulations! You've earned the right to dream big, to set yourself the goal of becoming not just a novelist but one successful enough to make her living solely from writing books. You weren't to know that it would take twenty years; that one of your books would go to #1 in the UK Kindle chart in the run-up to Christmas and you'd finally be able to think: *I've done it.*

So, what could you have done differently, leaving aside events you couldn't change such as bereavement, or your husband having a career blip?

You did right to persist, to take three part-time jobs in the evenings so you could write while the kids were at school. Maybe chucking in one of those jobs to further your writing career and then not selling a story for eight months was tricky, but you never gave up. That's good. Editors and agents rarely knock on doors to see whether a struggling writer lives there. Authors have to keep writing and submitting (and submitting and submitting), reading magazines about writing and attending conferences and talks. They need to learn not just about writing, but about publishing, too.

For most of those twenty years you did anything writing-related to earn a fee. You sold short stories, articles, novels, serials, courses and writing how-to. You led writing workshops, judged competitions and appraised manuscripts. You just about scraped together a contribution to the household.

I have to point out, though, that when three separate agents showed interest in you, they weren't just being nice. Agents only show interest when they're interested. Could you have fostered their interest and turned it into something good? I think so. You had no way of knowing then that in 2015 you'd begin working with the most awesome agent who'd guide you to bestsellerdom via a major publisher, and that the results would be worth the wait.

Did you miss other opportunities? Like letting a promising situation with a big publisher drop because your existing publisher, independent and small, was horrified? Well…yes. Would you do that again? *No.*

> But did you enjoy your writing? Was it a compulsion; did you have stories spinning in your imagination every day and know you had to bring them to the page? Yes. Did it make you happy? Absolutely. Can you think of a better job than "author?" No.

Neither can I, the present-day Sue. I'm a bestseller, an award winner who makes her living writing novels. It's now twenty-five years since I sold that first short story, twenty-five years filled with hard work…but also with joy. Writing still makes me happy.

Best wishes,

Sue Moorcroft

"You did right to persist "

TO THE PERSON WHO IS STRUGGLING AT WORK,

Firstly, you are good at what you do. Say it out loud: "I am good at what I do."

Feels silly, doesn't it? Say it twice more: "I am good at what I do … I am good at what I do." A friend asked me to do this when I was struggling. I laughed down the phone, embarrassed. I repeated it once and felt foolish. When I said it the second time, I felt a lump in my throat. The third time I said it, I started to cry.

The culture in my workplace had left me feeling worthless and unconfident. Sometimes, as I drove into work, I fantasized about crashing into a wall so I would have a valid reason not to go in. I lay awake all night long, with racing thoughts and a pounding heart for company. During the day, I had a constant pain in my chest, my back ached, and I felt on high alert.

Colleagues whispered anxiously in the corridors about accidentally provoking a dressing down or even a sacking. People cried and others walked by, unsurprised and resigned.

Then one morning, I stopped on my journey to work. I parked my car on a bridge over a river that cut through the landscape. A chill wind pinched at my cheeks and pulled at my hair. I clenched the freezing metal of the bridge in my hands and gazed out onto the water. Throughout my life, the water of mountain streams and sandy seas has always calmed me at times of stress. When my eldest child was born, he was ill and cried all night unless my husband pushed his pram around the deserted 2am streets or I held him gently in a warm bath.

The river scene slowly came into focus, and I watched mists rise from the river and evaporate. I felt my head clear and my shoulders begin to relax. I was not powerless, I realized, I had choices. As I looked out over the water, two swans emerged from under the bridge and slowly floated down the river. I had the sense of perspective I needed. I left my job.

Slowly, I felt myself returning to who I had been before. My husband and children were delighted that I was no longer sad, resigned, and exhausted. Looking back, I was shocked by the toxic practices which were accepted by the other employees. Looking forward, it felt as though I could now do anything.

Months later, while filling up the kettle to make a coffee, I suddenly thought to myself: I feel happy. For the first time in years, I felt pure happiness, unclouded by fear and anxiety.

If your daily work or study affects your sleep and makes you feel continually anxious, sad or depressed, remember that you have choices. It takes courage to decide to move on, especially when you feel unconfident and insecure, but what is the alternative? You are good enough and you deserve those moments of joy. Keep talking and try not to push away friends and family.

> I don't have regrets about what happened to me because I now notice all the tiny joyful things in each day.

I recognize that some people behave cruelly because they feel this is the only way. Ultimately, I'm glad I made the most important investment of all – an investment in my wellbeing.

I urge you to stop. Stand in a forest, on the street, in the garden, and think. Think about who you are and what you could be. You're good at what you do.

With love,

Sarah

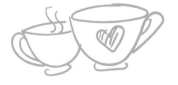

DEAR FRIEND,

My name is Chris Paterson. I served for seven years in the Argyll and Sutherland Highlanders (British Army) infantry, and I was medically discharged in 1998 after a serious ankle injury which required surgery in 1997. I did scaffolding for a few years until a serious accident caused me to be diagnosed with severe PTSD in May 2015. The accident triggered things I'd seen in my military career. After my accident, I struggled with anxiety, depression, flashbacks, nightmares, self-hate, suicidal thoughts every day, isolation, and anger.

I made a choice one day that I either had to go get help or not be here anymore, so I went to Combat Stress. They saved my life. They helped me understand what was going on in my head through therapy, both group and individual sessions with a psychiatrist.

I spent 14 weeks in total over a two-year period at their treatment center where they helped me with my sleep patterns, anxiety, self-hate, anger, and isolation.

They also put me in contact with a charity called the On Course Foundation (OCF). They are amazing. Through golf, they help serving military and veterans that have been injured, wounded or are sick.

Without this charity I definitely wouldn't be here today. They helped me get out the house to go to their events, which they hold all over the UK. One of the great things about these events is that there are like-minded veterans going through similar things as I was.

You weren't judged, just supported.

You also get the chance to meet some very special people/companies that want to support you on your new journey. People like Lewis Baker who works for American Golf. I met Lewis on one of my first events with OCF; he was at the event with the tour truck, showing us around it and helping us with new grips and giving us fantastic insight into how the pros get their clubs sorted for their events.

I went from not leaving the house, not living but just existing, to being able to compete in two Simpson cups. The Simpson Cup is an annual Ryder Cup styled tournament between teams of 13 injured servicemen and veterans from Great Britain and the USA.

My first was at St. Andrew's in 2019, and it was very special. I will remember the event for the rest of my life. Being the only Scottish player on the team in my home country and winning both my matches was unbelievable, especially when I think back and see myself in isolation at home, not able to go outside for months on end, and not even wanting to be here anymore.

The On Course Foundation charity, along with Combat Stress, has definitely changed my life. I still have bad days but they are now outweighed by the good days.

So, to anyone - especially a fellow veteran - reading my story and going through anything they are struggling with, please, go get help.

I know how hard it is to ask for help, but please don't suffer in silence.

Chris Paterson

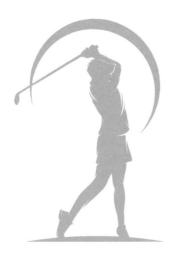

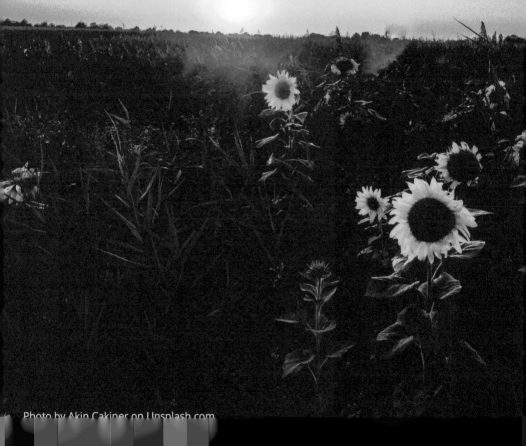

"It's never too late to face those fears and start living"

A LETTER TO MY 14-YEAR-OLD SELF,

Hey you!

I see you there, in that bed in the corner of the ward, headphones in with that blank expression. Your world is upside down. One minute you were a thirteen-year-old looking forward to her birthday, and by the end of that birthday you were in hospital. Three months later, you're still here. You're angry, confused, scared, alone and don't really know how to deal with it, but I'm here to tell you that it's going to be OK. It's 1989 and mental health isn't considered. You're doing the best you can with what you know right now – in fact, you're doing amazing, and I'm so proud of you. You've been through three lots of surgery, found out you have cancer, and had two weeks of radiotherapy so far, and you're only just 14 years old. On the outside, you're holding it together, but on the inside, I know your mind is a dark place.

I remember it well, like it was yesterday.

> But you know, Liz, you're going to cope. I'm not going to say it's going to be easy, but it's going to be OK.

You have so many adventures ahead of you and so many people to meet. You will fall in love and get your heart broken numerous times, but you'll have a family, a career and a normal life for a long time and there will be a period of your life where cancer is just a dark memory. You will be able to move on temporarily. However, you are going to have to face this one day – when you're ready, you will know, and once it's safe to look back, this will all make sense. I promise.

I want to say that this is your happy ending but you're going to need that strength for more cancer, surgery and finally chemo. Sorry, I know you think that not having chemo is a result at the moment. When you find out what sh*t that radiotherapy has done to your insides, you might temporarily wish you'd had no radiation.

I often think of you, sat on that bed. I remember the emotions so well, and I want to put my arms around you and tell you that you're safe, I'm with you. You have no idea how much you are facing alone, but I am so very proud of how you're coping, I know you've internalized it but that's OK for the moment. I have flashbacks of being in our corner, the curtain around my bed shut, the murmur from the ward clerk area as the night shift chattered, the heat of the ward – always roasting – and the hum of equipment around the bay. It fills me with fear and familiarity equally. A hospital ward should not become home to a teenager. But it did. And by accepting it, you begin to heal.

So, hang in there, girl. You've got so much to live for, and even though it takes you almost thirty years to heal, it's never too late to face those fears and to start living. One day you're going to be so proud of this story, and I'm holding your hand every step of the way.

I love you and I'm so proud of you.

Your 46-year-old self.

Liz

TO ANYONE WHO FEELS LOST –

I was an inquisitive 14-year-old, my parents were out, and what teenager never snooped through cupboards and drawers when they were alone in the house? What I found would have an impact on the rest of my life – my birth certificate with a different surname to the one I had. Who was I? Was I adopted? Did that mean my parents were not my parents? Was my brother not really my brother? Were my grandparents pretending to love me? A million questions scrambled my brain, and they were questions I wouldn't have the answers to for a further nine years.

I kept the discovery to myself, not wanting to unsettle the only family I knew, the only parents I knew to be my own, not wanting to know the truth. At 23, I had a mental breakdown. I had to give up my job, my flat, my stability – moving back to my family home to be cared for. Medication may have cured the physical effects of my illness, but mentally I knew I was being tortured by the constant invasion of thoughts around my birth certificate.

With help from a counsellor, I confronted my parents, and half my fears came true. The man who had brought me up, the man who was my "dad" was not my dad, my brother was not my full brother, my grandparents were not my grandparents, I was not who I thought I was.

This was such a difficult part of my life and still is to this day; the ramifications have been huge. There have been many years of discovery, both good and bad, a lot of hurt and sadness for those around me, my brother finding it hard to accept me and me wanting him to embrace and comfort me, which didn't happen for a long time, wondering why my parents never told me but all of this made me who I am today, a stronger, empathetic, honest (sometimes too honest!!) person. I, too, have my weaknesses, and those who know me understand my struggles with anxiety. It plagues me, and I loathe it, but if that is the only thing that I have to deal with as a result of my past, then I am grateful.

I now have two families, I gained two half-sisters, a half-brother, and another dad – don't get me wrong, there is still a lot of relationship-building to be done, but I know they are there for me.

The reason why I share this story is I want you to take positivity from it.

We all have issues and secrets that we carry with us throughout life, and they are nothing to be ashamed of – we learn from them, we gain from them, they enhance who we are, they challenge us, but most importantly they make us who we are, and I am thankful and accepting of who I am. I am still making discoveries.

Some days, weeks, and months I have my battles, still trying to make sense of it all, I get sad, angry, and lonely, but without those negative emotions, I would not appreciate the good and uplifting ones. We all know the saying, "Every cloud has a silver lining," and I can honestly say for me that this is true, my bond with the brother that I was brought up with is stronger than ever now, he is my sounding board, my best friend and he is my brother.

This is dedicated to my mum, who I lost to cancer five years ago. I want her to know that it was ok that she didn't tell me the truth, and I fully understand why – she was doing what every mum does for their children, trying to protect me, and I get that, I still have to find the courage to tell my own children this story, so I know how hard it was for you Mum. I love you xx

Amanda ♡

We all know the saying
'Every cloud has a
silver lining,' and I can
honestly say for me
THAT THIS IS TRUE

HELLO MY DARLING –

6 August 2021

Hello, my darling,

Many years ago you told me you were not the person I had grown to love, and that you had never really been that person, as for most of your life, you had been pretending.

I remember looking at you with tears in my eyes and saying, "If you are not that person – not the person I fell in love with – then I don't know if I can be with you."

You decided keeping me was worth more than being yourself, and so we never really discussed it again.

But I watched, over many years, as you struggled to live in the female form that was really not you. I looked on as you became more masculine, and I witnessed as many times you were shouted at or glared at for being in the female toilets. I saw you shrink into yourself, shoulders bent, hiding away from the world. You became a shell of yourself.

It became clear to me that I loved you enough to be with you no matter who you were. On that day, we started your transition. Eighteen years after that first conversation, an older, much wiser me came home from work one day and said, "Today is the day. Today is the day you really become your authentic self."

It has not been an easy journey, seeing you embark down a path that would forever change the outer form of you, one that I had loved for so long. But you did not love her, and that mattered to me.

As you started testosterone, I saw your features gradually change and hair begin to grow on your face and in places it had never been before. Then last year we travelled to London for your top surgery. That was the hardest day, for me, as a physical part of you I loved was removed. You came round from surgery elated, while I started a struggle with my innermost being, a struggle to come to terms with who I was, who I am and who I will be.

As an out lesbian activist for more years than I can say, I struggled to reconcile your transition with my identity. I had fought against Section 28 and campaigned for the right for us to legally marry as a same-sex couple. Who was I now? I remember being asked if your transition meant I was straight or bisexual and being so upset with the question because no, I was not either of those things. I felt angry at having to justify myself for loving you even through all the changes. Rejected by my lesbian peers as well as the straight community, I felt like I didn't fit in anywhere.

My beloved wife, after 21 years together, this is the day I thought would never come, the day when I have to say goodbye to you, and when you will disappear from my life forever. It's hard, but I have to do this. I have spent the last couple of years with you hovering in the corner of the room, always there in my peripheral vision, blocking out the amazing confident man you have become. To really open my heart to him, I have to let you go. I know that in saying goodbye I will open myself up to make way for my husband to come in.

I will never forget you, my dearest wife, and the time we had together. Those wonderful memories will forever remain with me. But I will walk on, hand in hand with my husband, to make new memories, and I will always be thankful to you for bringing us together.

> On our wedding cake, we had the words "I have found the one whom my soul loves - Song of Solomon 34." If that be the case, that our souls love each other, then what does it matter what that soul looks like?

So goodbye, my darling, sweetest wife and hello, my brave, beloved husband.

Your wife, then and now

Krystyna

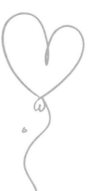

REFLECTIONS

DEAR WANDERER OF OUR WORLD,

Silence, loneliness, departure, death...

The most powerful answer to a question. The unknown, untold, absence, and in our modern times

ghost(ing).

Silence is seen as the end.

However, silence has the single most effective healing property.

It gives you time

Time to get to know who you are

Introspect

In peace and for your wellbeing.

Take a moment in the chaos – breathe

Dive into your values, what drives you – from your work to the dinner you cooked, or the lines you

write before going to sleep.

Find yourself

How you connect with nature, feelings, sleep – how you appreciate small things, the sound of food sizzling, birds in the parks, water by the sea, and your own heartbeat.

Make silence great again!

For all the over-thinkers, lost, clarity seekers, and curious souls embracing silence can become your

secret weapon, use it wisely

From someone who had to build themselves back on their own

Anonymous

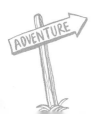

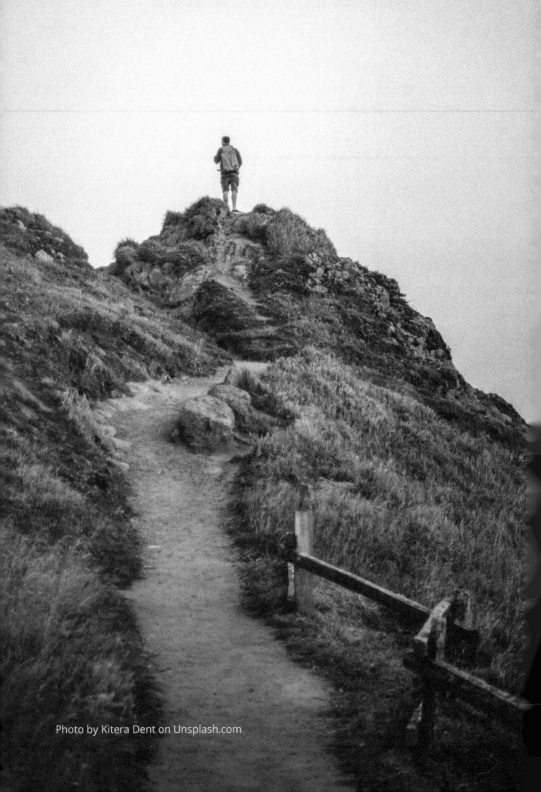

DEAR READER,

Hardship comes in many forms, and we all experience these throughout our life - it is very much a component of the human experience.

Sometimes knowing this alone can provide us with solace and reassurance and can bind us together with others in a form of almost global citizenship. I hope this and the remainder of the letter provides you with the reassurance that you are not alone and that there is always a path to overcoming adversity, no matter how far off the beaten track it may be.

When asked to contribute a letter to this wonderful project I contemplated about what I could write about. I, like all humans, have faced adversity in various forms, but the nature of my own personal hardships and the kind of challenges I face during my time on this Earth have undoubtedly been cushioned due to the hardships my parents endured, allowing me to take my place in a very different world to the one they experienced growing up.

So, I've decided to adopt the role of storyteller and share with you the story of two rather remarkable humans, to both capture determination, resilience and aspirations personified but also to offer a small token of our (mine and my siblings') appreciation of our parents' unstoppable will.

The story begins with the coming together of two lives – a young man, from New Delhi, recently graduated from The University of Delhi and a young woman born in Tanzania but raised in England by a widowed mother of five children. Both from humble beginnings, the two met and were married in the autumn of 1976. Together they endeavored to build a life in England, away from their original country of origin, a life that would go beyond their own experiences.

In the graphic novel, *The Arrival* by Shaun Tan (and I would highly recommend you get hold of a copy!), Tan depicts the journey of two immigrants and the alien language and lifestyle they find themselves

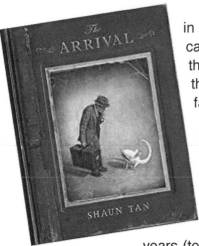

in upon moving to a foreign land. The pictures captured in this book, offer a window into the life that awaited my parents as they embarked on the journey of a lifetime, leaving their friends, family, and countries behind.

Upon arriving to England, my mother and father sought employment and secured roles in factory work and in the postal service, respectively. In 1983, the first of their four children were born, my eldest brother arrived in 1984, my youngest brother an exact ten years (to the day) after my parents were married and me, in 1990. My mother left work and embarked on a full-time role as a homemaker. Her days were consumed with school runs, nursery drop-off and pick-ups, household chores and cooking, as well as entertaining four children, each with unique and very distinct personalities and interests.

My sister loved reading, my brothers' sports, and I, singing and dancing. The living room was a concoction of sports equipment, reading books, artwork, and endless noise (how I best describe my melodic expressions at the time).

Meanwhile, my father worked tirelessly for 24 years at the Royal Mail, first sorting post and eventually driving large lorries of post cross-country, often averaging 90-hour weeks. Despite this, we never felt his absence and he always remained present and supportive in our education, interests, and thoughts.

When I recently questioned, "So that must have been really exhausting, right Dad?" he responded, "Exhausting, yes – but incredibly enjoyable too. I was devoted to my work and if I had to do it all over again … I would." Similarly, when I asked my mother how difficult it must have been to raise 4 children of varying ages whilst Dad worked every hour possible, she also remarked, "I used to love it."

If having one determined, diligent, and devoted parent was a blessing … our blessings as children were doubled. Two individuals from different walks of life, coming together with a mutual sense of work ethic, resilience and stick-to-iteveness (that Simpsons reference is for you, dear brothers) to craft the conditions to enable my siblings and me to achieve our dreams and aspirations. All graduates, all able to pursue a better life and all humbled by the sacrifices our parents made in the past to pave the way for our present day.

Thank you, Mum and Dad, for so beautifully and eloquently modelling what fortitude looks like in action and I hope that this letter crystalizes and celebrates YOUR achievements and your remarkable journey.

Lekha Sharma

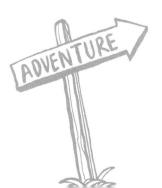

TO ANYONE FACING THE WORST —

"There is no evidence to suggest that chemotherapy will work, his quality of life may be limited, his mobility will be seriously impaired, and his brain may not develop beyond that of a new-born baby. You need to consider palliative care." There it was, the moment as a parent you never want to experience. You are going to have to let your son go.

Our boy came into this world in October 2019 and a month later after deteriorating to the point where he was screaming uncontrollably, refusing to feed and sleeping 20 hours a day we took him to A&E. Here he was diagnosed with a brain tumor the size of two oranges. Two oranges, in the skull of a 4-week-old baby. Whisked to Leeds General Infirmary within hours of arriving at our local A&E we were plunged into the greatest and most dreadful fight of our lives. Roux was that poorly neither of us could go in the ambulance with him, he needed that much equipment to keep him alive – he was on the brink of death.

Arriving at Leeds General Infirmary we were informed by a doctor that he was incredibly ill and there was a "serious chance we would lose him." Crying into my dad's chest, I screamed and screamed "Dad, I cannot lose him, I cannot lose him, I cannot lose him," over and over again. They'd already began an operation on him to relieve the pressure on his brain and we didn't even see him whilst we sat in Leeds A&E.

> I lost myself that night, it's a blur - I must have
> sat in that waiting room with my head in my hands
> sobbing for eight hours straight.

When the surgeon came through to see us, I expected the worse, but how wrong I was to think like that. Roux is a warrior – he was not going to give in.

The following three months involved surgery after surgery, living at the hospital away from our other son who stayed with grandparents whilst my wife and I held our tiny little man's hand as he lay on a hospital bed. Tumor debulking every few days, marathon surgeries one after the other, fingers crossed and gripping each other hoping that more of the tumor had been removed each time. 10%, 23%, 33% - slowly but surely our surgeon was removing this disease from our little man's brain. Each time, Roux would come out in a terrible state: his poor little body scarred and swollen.

Then it happened, Roux took a turn on intensive care, he was losing blood, brain fluid and his oxygen levels had plummeted. Roux was worked on the ward to try and stabilize him, but it wasn't looking good – he'd need emergency surgery just hours after his last tumor removal surgery. He got through it – of course he did, but then came the conversation we were dreading. "Roux isn't handling surgery well, surgery is no longer an option, and you need to consider palliative care. We will make him comfortable."

We spoke to the nurse who was looking after Roux on the High Dependency Unit after we had that conversation with the doctors, and she says how our words when we came back have stuck with her: "How can we let our boy fight as hard as he had so far to still be here to then give up on him?"

We would let him fight. Fight he did.

Roux got stronger and stronger in the coming weeks. His movement was improving, he fed better, and he started to smile. We had our boy. Every day we could see him making progress and when the surgeon came to us to say he'd be taking him to surgery again, we broke down in delight. Madness. Celebrating that your child would go through another huge brain surgery is quite something. But the other option was unimaginable. Roux went on to have surgery and more tumor was removed. We were nearly there.

MRIs and CT scans were just regular life now. Sitting waiting for a call to see if the tumor is growing again makes you sick to the pit of your stomach. One of those calls revealed that the tumor was growing back – another surgery.

Roux's had 11 brain surgeries in total now but as it stands at the moment is tumor-free. Roux is two years old now and says a few words, eats on his own, holds his bottle, gives us kisses and cuddles and smiles from ear to ear every day. The fight in him is greater than anything I've ever known. Each morning I wake up and cannot wait to see his smiling face – a face that at one point we were convinced that we would be burying.

I just do not see life the same way anymore, I cherish every moment: laying with him in a morning at 5.45am whilst he chugs his milk; the Saturday mornings walking back from his brother's football training in the pram; the forty minutes playtime on the carpet after work before tucking him into bed and the bath time splashes.

> These are the things that matter in this world. Love.
> Nothing else does - it really, really doesn't.

This boy is the bravest and strongest little man in the world and I'm so incredibly proud to call him my son. What he has done to be here still is utterly beyond belief. Of course, there are challenges ahead, he is suffering from seizures, is yet to walk and is clearly at least a year developmentally behind children of his age. This does not matter one bit though, he's happy, healthy and most importantly here. Roux was put on this earth for a reason, and he's been kept on this earth to do something special in the future too. Fight on little man – this life has been one worth fighting for.

Antony Owen

Roux's privileged father, writing from the High Dependency Unit in Hull Royal Infirmary (17.10.2021)

EVERY TIME

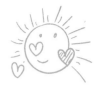

Sometimes you walk a path you didn't expect

But you'd choose that way every time again

The pain, the trauma, the damn right misery

But it's all worth it, because you're still with me

You fought and battled with true courage in your heart

Giving in wasn't an option, there's no way you'd depart

Watching you suffer, wasn't fair – the world's cruel

But we knew of your strength; we believed in you

Now my eyes swell instead with tears of pure pride

That smile and that grin are building me back inside

Those vile hours and days are slowly starting to fade

Replaced with your joy and better memories are made

Sometimes you walk a path you didn't expect

But you'd choose that way every time again.

By Antony Owen (Roux's father)

DEAR FRIENDS,

"Live your life without regret. It's complicated, it's challenging and shorter than you can ever imagine, but you must find the smallest of reasons every day to make it truly wonderful."

My Nanna was called Hetty, and these were her words, words I have held onto like priceless fragments of life. I have lived another 35 years since she whispered this to me, not long before she passed. I miss my Nanna enormously, but this gift of words has been a comfort through the ups and downs of my life, and I hope by sharing her wisdom she can hold onto your hand and guide you too.

This is what I know of living.

- Dream big, nothing is impossible.
- Be yourself, you never know who you are inspiring.
- Admire the path of others but always follow your own.
- Embrace your uniqueness.
- Your imperfections are your beauty.
- Say no if saying yes isn't for you.
- Be kind, even to your enemies. If nothing else, it will disturb them beyond belief.
- The older you become, the less you will care what anyone else thinks.
- If you worry you don't fit in, please don't, your tribe will find you.
- Look after your body, it's more precious than you realize.
- If a library is your happy place, enjoy the story, I'm with you.
- Look up at the sky and breathe deeply every day.
- Success doesn't look the same for everyone.

You can only fail if you don't try.

- You will be OK, I promise.

Love *Hetty & Paula*

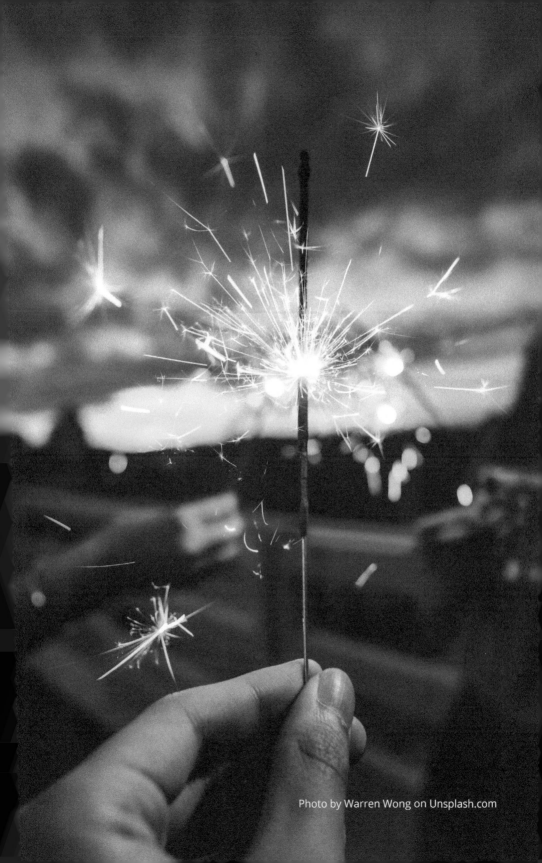

REMEMBER

These onion days ache,

force tears, unshed, peel back your

skin to tenderness

below. Even onions are

sweet in the right conditions

By *Cate Haynes*

TO ANYONE FEELING PRESSURED TO BE SUCCESSFUL –

Positioned at the right-hand corner of my father's desk, was a poem by Robert Chambers carefully torn from a magazine. The words and paper had faded from the many years of being under glass, but the clipping stood out for its significance as the only piece of paper on an otherwise empty and neat desktop.

My father, a retired surgeon – a self-described "country doctor" – and a servant to his community, is a hardworking, thoughtful, humble man and not one for platitudes or showmanship. By all accounts, he remains a pilar of the community and continually sets the bar high for his family and those around him.

It was surprising then when I first read the poem. Surprising not for what the poem communicated, but rather what the poem represented. Of all the motivational and relevant poems out there, what is it about this poem that struck my father that he would carry this with him for his entire career?

Perhaps this Robert Chambers poem was a reminder of what he had become and that while his time has passed as a highly successful physician, when people look back and assess his overall contribution, it is not so bad that he has become a has-been.

Many children of successful parents feel the overwhelming pressure of being more successful than their parents. Most, however, don't succeed. I don't think I will ever surpass my father in character, prestige or standing, but I also recognize that I still have the potential to be a *could be, an are*, and hopefully *a has-been*.

> I'd rather be a could be if I could not be an are. For a could be has a chance for reaching par.

But I'd rather be a has-been than a might-have-been by far. For a might-have-been has never been, but a has-been was once an are.

Sincerely,

Bill Hughes

To WHOEVER IS READING THIS,

No, I'm not picking that up … It's not because I don't want to, it's because I CAN'T!

What do you mean it's broken? Is it still broken? I don't understand. Can I still do everything that I want?

I have been told a few times how lucky I am, but none of those compare to the day I was told that I was lucky to still be walking. I broke my back in two places playing a game that I loved and will never play again. A momentary lapse in concentration, a surge of adrenaline and a stubbornness to continue saw me fight through a white-hot flash of pain. Not wanting to let others down, I carried on.

Nobody knew I had broken my back. It wasn't until eight months later that eventually an eagle-eyed doctor spotted the repaired bones. Luckily it was just the bone but being told time and time again that there was nothing wrong with me and that it was just a sore muscle became so frustrating and infuriating and demoralizing.

I have never experienced pain like that in my life. Being unable to sit, or stand, or lie down for long periods for months on end can really wear down your spirit. I lost count of how many tears I shed. Being told that it was, in fact, broken came as such a relief. I just needed a reason for the pain.

Pain can overwhelm you. It can change your personality. It can change who you are. It affects your loved ones. It affects your way of life. It affects the decisions you make. And the decisions you don't make. It throws you into dark places that are hard to get out of.

If you let it.

I didn't let it. I did bend down to pick it up. Every single time. I put my body through the most excruciating pain, but I bent down, and I picked it up.

Sometimes it's just so easy to take the easy way. Something as simple as dropping something on the floor and choosing to leave it there because it's a lot easier than bending over.

Dealing with pain all day every day is draining. When I open my eyes every day, I know what's in store for me and I know that I have a few choices that I can make. I have a two-year-old little girl that is my world, and I have the most supportive wife a man can ask for. So, the first decision I make is for them. I decide to get up with a smile and show my little girl that her dad can roll around and play with her and have a picnic with her on the bathroom floor. If she wants me to stand up ten times to get the imaginary peanut butter and bananas, then that's what I do. If she wants me to run around like a stinky skunk, then for those few minutes I am a stinky skunk. I am there for her because I have put my mind in charge. I have made the choice. I so badly want to be her hero. I want to be the dad that can kill the dragon and scare away all the monsters. I want to be the dad that she is proud of.

> And I don't want to let my wife down. She is the
> one and only person for me, so I can't let her down
> because I am in pain. They are my family and my
> whole world.

Pain lives with me every day. I know that I will never be better, and I know there are limitations to the things that I can do, but I also know what a positive mindset can achieve. I have had to work so hard at it, and admittedly some days are easy, and some days are hard. Some days are really hard. I often get told, "I don't know how you do it." The simple answer is because I have to. I dread to think what things would be like if I didn't. I have built an incredible mental strength towards it and have a habitually positive attitude towards things because it makes things so much easier for me. It doesn't happen overnight, but you know what, it does happen.

My positive mindset has driven me to challenge myself to do things that ordinarily I wouldn't do. It's a way of showing myself and others that it is possible to do things when it gets a bit tough. A way of proving that what should be an excuse is actually a motivation. I am a marathon runner, not because I love running, or because I am an athlete, but because I challenged my mind to drag my body around a 26-mile route when my body didn't want to do it. Soon I will row a boat across the Atlantic Ocean. Not because I am a rower but because my mind will tell my body that it needs to fall in line and get the job done.

These are extreme cases and challenges. But they are my challenges which my mind will overcome. Your challenge may be to bend down to pull your socks on, or to walk to the shop instead of drive, or to talk in front of a room full of people. Whatever it may be, whether it's a physical challenge, an emotional challenge or just your own confidence, put your mind in charge. What's easy for some may be difficult for others so don't compare, don't use other people as a benchmark. Do it for yourself. Do it because you want to do it. Do it because it's difficult. But do yourself and your loved ones a favor … do it.

I try and live by a very simple saying. I find that it gets me through a lot of difficult physical challenges and motivates me to just keep going and I hope that it does the same for you.

"One day I won't be able to do this.
Today is not that day."

Take care of yourself and your loved ones,

Darryl Thole

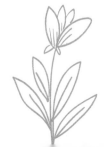

TO ANYONE WHO NEEDS TO FIND BEAUTY

There is no such thing as a discernable "happy ending" waiting at the end of a season or a transition, at least for some of us. Sometimes the happy ending is merely pockets of light breaking through. It's the discovery of glimmers of beauty tucked within your storyline. In real life, a fairytale ending is in the telling of my story, bringing healing to your story.

I was planning to enjoy a relaxing evening watching the sunset on Lake Shasta, but as I looked through my patio window just beyond the trees, I saw a billowing pillar of snow-white smoke striping the blue sky. In California, the prolonged summer droughts turn the entire state into a tinderbox, and for the past 10 years, the state has been trying to burn itself to the ground. So, it will be no surprise if, over the next 10 years, every part of the state will have burned. As a result of this fire frequency, the ability to read smoke signals becomes second nature.

I knew this was a definite sign of the beginning of a wildfire; I hoped for the best and turned in for the night. However, I was awakened the following day to the sound of air tankers flying low overhead and the detonation of propane tanks attached to homes. The pillar of flame transformed into a raging wildfire, and due to the location, the firetrucks were unable to get to it. The only way to fight it was by air and by day only, which meant that the fire would continue to grow by night! Before it was said and done, it would have taken thirteen 1200-gallon air tankers, 8 helicopters, 180 engines, 12 bulldozers, 22 water tenders, and over 1600 personnel and crew to contain what is now known as the Fawn Fire.

I felt very unprepared. My mind was inundated with what-if questions. What if we ran out of gas? What if everyone was trying to take the same route out of town? What if panicked drivers caused an accident? What if the smoke overtakes us and we can't breathe? What if the fire jumped ahead of us and blocked the road? Can I drive through a wall of flames and not crash? Soon the sun would be darkened, and morning would be night. I wondered if I had the courage to run through a wall of fire or lie on the cement while a fire tornado takes wing, cutting off my escape. These scenarios were actual accounts of those who fled the most destructive fire in California in a century, The Camp Fire of 2018. Suddenly my breathing started to get shallower, and I could feel a panic attack peeking in through the threshold of my heart.

The only thing I could think to do was go outside. I was immediately met with smoldering embers and leaves raining from the sky. Suddenly, the vibrancy of the colors was heightened before my eyes. Every surface seemed to have been enhanced by computer-generated imagery. Even with the fire bearing down on the city, I forgot to be afraid. These were pigments I never knew existed.

What a strange sight I must have been, standing in the road, grinning like a bobcat during a blizzard of ash and debris laced with fire. Above were heavy grayish and brown clouds of smoke hanging across the blue sky like window valances. Trailing right behind were 70-foot flames curtaining the sky, burnt orange and red off in the distance. For some reason, I couldn't help but be in awe at how beautiful all the colors were. It all felt surreal. After brushing the ash from my hair and clothes, I finally went inside and sat at the dining room table, playing with the burned leave that had drizzled around my feet. A realm of beauty than can only be seen in a storm.

Please be gracious with me. I realized how farcical this all sounds. I would have never seen this type of beauty were it not for this suffocating darkness that enveloped the city. I will never trivialize hardship but would you please wander with me? Please dare to wonder what beauty is waiting to be found amid the teary-eyed blindness of your pain, while choking on the shock of your hardship or through the smog of a seemingly never-ending conflict. What's being highlighted just beyond the firestorm of life?

What gems are waiting for you to place
in the treasure chest called your story?

Anonymous

" I couldn't help but be in awe of how beautiful all the colors were "

ENDLESS WORLDS
By Alya Oliver

I always feel restless

And how could I not

When the world is endless

Filled with secrets

That are waiting to be unlocked

Please honey don't waste your life

Worrying about the disapproval

From other people's eyes

People can sometimes be cruel

But stop believing in their lies

And then the true you shall arise

To ANYONE SEEKING SOLACE –

Everything is sacred. EVERYTHING. Is sacred.

Be grateful for every. Single. Precious. Moment.

…because it will never be the same again, nothing lasts forever.

Love is an ENDLESS flow. Give and receive freely. The more you give, the more you have.

Pause often and *re-member*. Embody the moment and find present awareness. Give gratitude before all else.

Seek solace and wisdom in the quiet silence of the trees. Watch how they stand rooted and flow freely in their branches. They are the elders. Listen to their wisdom.

Life is a mandala of ever-unfolding beauty and changes continually.

Trust that the fluctuations have structure and holds perfection if we are able to let go…

Never cling, grip or attach. Life is not meant to stay stagnant. It is an ever-flowing river of experience. Do not grasp hold so tightly you miss the subtle messages, the beauty, joy and peace.

There is huge power and potency in the silence, in the subtle, in the pause. Nature reconnects us back in with that subtle stream of pulsing consciousness. Do not underestimate the power of subtlety.

Nature is medicine. Plants are medicine. Your mind is limited to its belief systems, to its programming, to its upbringing. Allow the plants to show you where you can grow and expand.

You cannot save anyone. Only we can save ourselves. But we can, and we must, hold space in unconditional love and non-judgmental support for each other. Community is what is lacking and where we have gone wrong. It has never been about competition or greed.

Do not let greed rule you or confuse you. Give first but be open to receive. You are abundant by nature.

Be vulnerable. Be real. Be honest. Communicate. Listen. Feel your feelings. Don't try to fix anything, it's already perfect. That includes you.

Kristen

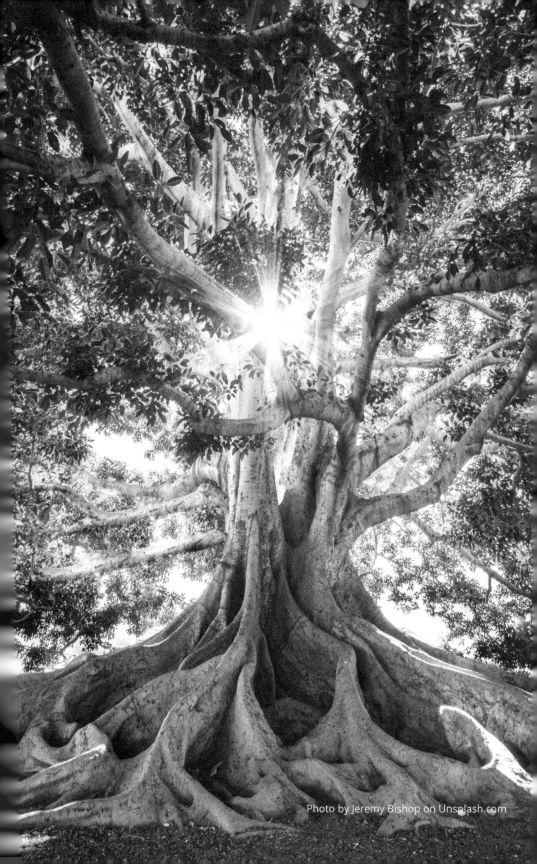

TO ANYONE WONDERING ABOUT HINDSIGHT –

I never understood the essence of what hindsight was until I experienced it, the term is often used as a throwaway comment – "upon hindsight." I want to share the hardest lesson that consumed me for years but if I had been equipped with what I know now, perhaps I wouldn't have to use that very same terminology. When I use it, it's really me talking about the red flags that were missed as well as the subtle signs before those came along.

In 2008, I was in my second year of university, had started a job to help with the costs of living, and was pretty settled in my routine. I had made some great friends in my new place of work and one of them had taken a liking to me. At first, I thought they were just over-complimentary but looking back, that's clearly not the case. Things moved fast between us. We were going out together in our friendship circle, enjoying each other's company and having fun.

Suddenly, we were in a relationship together and I can see the subtle signs that are my "upon hindsight" moments. Plans with my friends being changed because he hadn't seen me all day and wanted to spend time with me. The jealous moments on a night out when other men looked my way. His ex-girlfriend calling around his house asking for him back and him calling her crazy.

It never crossed my mind that he would harm me. I believed he was in love with me, and no one had ever loved me so strongly like this before.

We moved in together and I fell pregnant and had to defer my final year at university. My pregnancy was almost like his guarantee that I was his. Things progressed from the subtle signs to giving me ultimatums, waking me up in the night to accuse me of cheating on him, making me sleep on the floor as he was disgusted with me, not allowing me to meet up with my mum alone, cutting me off from friends. I was 20 years old, 110 miles away from home and feeling like there was no escape.

I married him, had a second child and was stuck in a never-ending cycle for years. I thought the problem was with me; I tried to prevent arguments by conforming to how he would like me to run things in the house. I didn't have many friends left, I didn't visit my family, I spent as little as I could to avoid going into more debt, I stopped working because he couldn't manage the kids on his own. He would pick out what I wore and buy my clothes – and I am just skimming the surface. But there was nothing I could do because it was never going to be good enough.

> There were a hundred reasons to leave and a thousand to stay.

I did manage to escape after several years of trying to be the best wife, the best mum, the best homemaker I could be. It took me a while, but I learned that this was a form of domestic abuse – it wasn't all about physically hurting someone. I also learnt that the abuse doesn't end when the relationship does, not just with post-abuse but with the sub-conscience he had given me. It has taken several years for me to find my feet and put the tools in place to help recover from the coercive control I was subjected to.

I never completed my university degree, but thankfully I can use my lived experiences to help others understand what emotional abuse can look like. That the "upon hindsight" feeling that hurts me greatly is something that can be shared, from subtle signs to red flags. No one deserves to be groomed into an unhealthy relationship and be left to feel there is no way out. Look for the subtle signs, take things slow and find healthy relationships that make you flourish.

Jennifer Gilmour
Author & Advocate

If I had the opportunity, I'd like to send a letter to my younger self. The 20-something year old full of anxiety and empty of confidence.

Perhaps on the days you lack confidence or self-belief, these words will help you like I know they would have me.

DEAR JERI,

There is a lot we can't control but I want you to know you do have choices available to you. We can make small choices moment to moment within each day. Even in our most constricted situations, we have a choice.

I want you to know the world isn't as scary as you think. It isn't as out of reach as you believe, and there is unexpected joy in life that you could never imagine.

I've made a list of what I have learnt and wish you knew …

Science and spirituality are both valid.

To notice that I am simply alive makes me grateful to make the most of it.

Co-creation is better than hierarchy.

I am ok even when I feel like I am not. I am ok.

Saying no is a skill that needs to be mastered.

Stopping and slowing down is an achievement.

Feminine and masculine energy both exist within us with equal importance.

Therapy is more than I imagined.

Love isn't what I expected.

Anxiety can be controlled.

Emotional intelligence is more helpful than IQ.

Meditation works but I will forget to do it.

Natural parenting is life changing.

Asking for help can make others feel useful.

Being dyslexic doesn't mean you can't be an academic.

Set emotional boundaries. It makes people in your life feel safe and trust you.

A long exhalation calms the body.

It's never about the huge changes – it's always about the 1% improvements.

Manifesting works.

And never justify yourself to anyone. Ever.

Listen more. Speak up with your ideas. Ask questions. Ask for help. Take calculated risks.

And save a little bit of money each month, no matter how small!

Jerilee Claydon

Clinical Psychotherapist UKCP, MBACP

Parenting educator

Newborn observation Practitioner

"Sunrise came as a golden tunnel to a world of forever light"

TO ANYONE THINKING OF ENDING –

The morning after I ended it all, I woke up. I ate toast and drank tea.

The morning after I ended it all, I fell in love.

I fell in love with my mother who sat in my old bedroom caressing my personal belongings until it was cold and dark.

I fell in love with my father who read my note over and over.

I fell in love with my daughter who once believed in unicorns, but now sat at her desk in school trying desperately to believe I still existed.

The morning after I ended it all, sunrise came as a golden tunnel to a world of forever light.

The morning after I ended it all, I tried to un-end it all, but this was not possible.

K Dillon

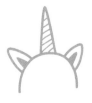

To My Older Self,

There's nothing wrong with me,

I'm as healthy as can be.

I have arthritis in both knees,

when I talk, it's with a wheeze.

I'm overweight, can't get thin,

but I'm awfully well for the shape that I'm in.

Sleep is denied me night after night,

but every morning I find I'm alright.

My memory's failing,

my head's in a spin,

but I'm awfully well for the shape that I'm in.

The moral of this tale as it unfolds,

is that all of us are growing old.

We often say that we're fine, with a grin,

rather than let people know the shape that we're in.

Karen Dillon

TO MY DEAREST CHILDREN,

Am I even allowed to address you like that? Society, after all, now considers you adults, but you will always be my children. Adulthood has transformed our relationship in subtle and not so subtle ways. What was previously parental guidance now sometimes feels like interference; yet, as a parent, I need an outlet to share life's lessons, our family's collective subconscious, and any wisdom that might protect you from pain.

So, I cannot help but write these letters and hope
that in a moment of search or solitude or loneliness
they may find your open heart to receive the love
they contain.

Let's start at the beginning. One of my earliest childhood memories that did not involve my parents was my second day of kindergarten at the Aga Khan School in Tanzania, the first time we were allowed on the playground. We wore green uniforms with new Oxford shoes. I ran out with all the kids into the sweltering heat, free from the stress of the class. I was about to approach a girl with interesting hair to ask her to be my friend when a boy told me that I could never climb the jungle gym because I was a girl. My competitive streak, strong even in those young years, propelled me up the structure, the boy on the other side, taunting me. Three steps up and I slipped, falling to the ground. Bleeding, all I wanted was my father to come and take me into his arms, while striking the ground and scolding it for hurting me. As I swallowed back my tears, more from embarrassment than pain, five girls ran towards me. One started to help me up, the other caressed my head and wiped the dirt from my uniform, the third offered me a lollipop straight from her mouth (which I gladly accepted--times were simpler then), the fourth stood guard and pushed back the boys who had gathered nearby, laughing at my plight, and the fifth asked if she should get the teacher. Within a few moments, I was playing again and had a collection of new friends.

As I reflect on this memory, I am aware that the girls who showed me those small acts of kindness became my friends but not ones I have today – we parted ways when I moved to Canada 2 years later. That incident gave me life skills that have helped me thrive wherever life has taken me. I learned that it requires strength to accept help. The universe will give you what you need but you have to be open to accept it. The help did not come in the form I was expecting, but it came in a better form for the future me. Each girl helped in her own way. Human instinct is to be of service to one another. It helps us with our purpose and happiness.

Since that day, many years ago, I have consciously tried to help people in small ways – from a smile to everyone I meet; to making faces at babies to get them to laugh – the pure sound of joy; to spending time with the elderly listening to their stories, especially when those who once did are no longer in their lives. Small acts that take up the vibrational energy of everyone involved and through inertia set in motion with these small acts, karma slowly shows us a more promising future. Having practiced this for decades, there are two keys to make it a success. First, always come from a place of gratitude, the fuel that makes those small acts resonate. Second, remember that the first place for the kind act is with you.

> Why not give that first smile to yourself first thing
> in the mirror? Your smiles were always the best part
> of my day.

Love Always,

Xoxo *Mom*

This is an extract from letters written by Shemin Nurmohamed, called the Karma of Kindness to her children when they left for university.

DEAR MOTHER,

Thank you for looking after us so well,
One little boy and one little girl.
We held your hand, you gave us your heart.
You certainly gave us a wonderful start.

Until parenthood came, little did I know,
The day-to-day chores that helped us to grow.
Mums are taken for granted, I realize now,
The cooking, the cleaning, the cheek of us – wow!

The journey to school, the weekly clubs.
Gosh – the amount that you did to look after us.
The stories at bedtime, the rush in the morning,
I now joke to friends: children should come with a warning.
Throughout all the chaos, come bundles of love.
A cuddle in bed, a kiss from above.
You helped us to read, you taught us to write,
But oh, were we grateful? No, we'd give you a fright.

Eye rolling, tantrums, a little bit of cheek.
Mother knew best, seven days of the week.
You dressed us so well, from top to toe.
You took us to places we wanted to go.

You plaited my hair, you cleaned football boots,
You became the tooth fairy, when we lost a tooth.

Trips to the doctors, some to A & E,
Truly our hero, the best you could be.

Our greatest critic and strongest adviser,
Giving us words, that made us both wiser.
I bet sometimes you thought "please give me a rest."
When all you were doing, was trying your best.

I now look up; to the moon and the stars,
Seeking your guidance, and comfort from afar.
Believe me I listened to every word you had to say,
Your kindness and strength is now paving the way.

You encouraged us to realize our true desire,
An angel above, whom we truly admire.
Upon reflection, I appreciate everything you did,
I wish I had done so, when I was a kid.

Lots of love,

Lou

Xxx

By Louise Bunyan, in memory of our Mum,
Margaret Grant Irvine Bunyan, who lost her battle to cancer
in May 2021.

TO ANYONE DEALING WITH MENTAL HEALTH –

"What do you know about mental health!" he said
The same question once popped into my head
Because I sometimes felt bad
That I wasn't quite as mad
As those who had cried, screamed or bled

But ill health of the mind can be ever so silent
If behaves like this so you become compliant
With social norms
And the need to conform
but ignoring its existence makes it more violent

So put on the kettle and make some tea
Wait for it to brew and then later breathe
There is no shame
In not being the same
As those who need more sugar than me

We experience poorly heads in different ways
"It's all relative" is an important phrase
Be kind to your feelings
It'll help with your healing
So, you know how to cope with rainier days

Tilly Humphreys

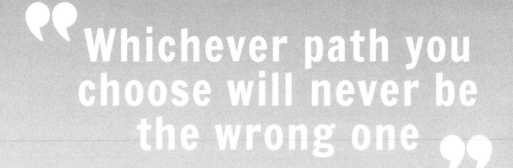

"Whichever path you choose will never be the wrong one "

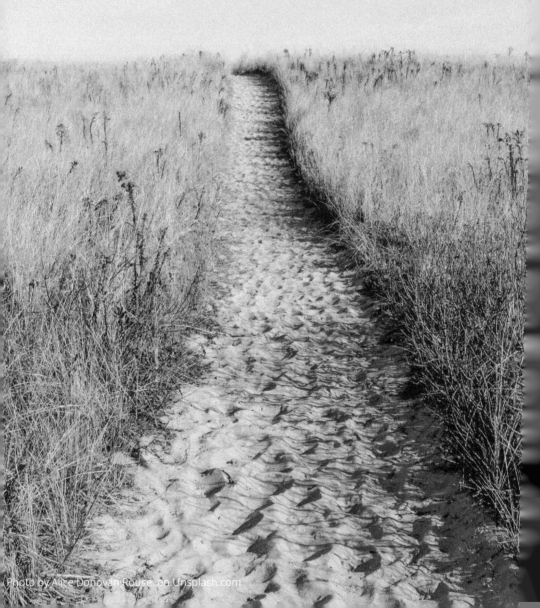

DEAR YOUNGER S.J.,

Firstly, I want to tell you how much I love you.

I'm fifty-seven now and am wiser and more experienced about life.

So, these are some of the important things I've learned during my journey and want to pass on to you.

There are times when you will need to speak up and be heard, but there are also times when you will need to keep quiet and listen to what others have to say.

It's fine to push yourself out of your comfort zone. Too much self-doubt is not healthy but having some self-doubt will push you to do better and try harder.

> Life is one big learning curve; you will never be too old to learn, and I am still learning every single day.

Always remain curious, try to look at things from other people's perspectives as well as your own.

There will always be occasional bumps on the road of life, but that's all they are. You will always return to level ground.

Believe in yourself.

Talent alone does not bring success; hard work and effort pays off in the long term.

Life will give you lots of choices. Whichever path you choose will never be the wrong one; even failures are lessons learned.

Make sure you always make time for the people you love.

Worrying over something won't solve your problems but taking direct action will.

Always forgive and try to understand why the person you are forgiving took the action they did.

Speak aloud; never be afraid to voice your opinion as long as your words are said with integrity, and never allow anyone to bully you.

Your career and your journey through life are your own, and although you may wish to share it with a partner, your journey will always be your own.

Always be honest to others and to yourself. Only work in a job that you have a passion for, unless you need money to pay the bills and buy food.

Care about how other people see you, but don't live by other people's standards, only your own.

Aspire to always do better than you did the day before.

Make every day count, remembering that it may be your last.

Surround yourself with kind, genuine people, and recognize toxic, negative people for who they really are.

Remember that love is more than passion, romance and candles.

Try to help others whenever possible.

Be grateful every day for the small pleasures life has to offer you.

Laugh and sing joyfully at every opportunity.

Try to be sensible with money and always remember those less fortunate than yourself.

I wish you a life full of fun, hopes and dreams coming true.

With Love,

S.J. Gibbs (Your older self)

To ANYONE WHO WANTS TO FIND JOY —

Some days feel like moments, weeks like days,
months pass by like years and years seem like yesterday.

So much growth yet still the same.
Ever-changing, always unchanged.

Memories of past moments; a year full of surprise.
Surrender to the moment – all is well; dry your eyes.

What's gone will always be part
of the person that stands here today.

Fragments of people, places, sunshine and rain.

Letting go of the past, the future.
I reside here and now.

Photos hold the remnants of a time gone by,
a time I long for right here and right now.

Sadness doesn't need to stay long
as I am certain of the beauty that lays ahead.

For now, I will smile, as I wait
to see you again.

Anonymous

To My Undercover Hero –

No, this hero does not have a cap, nor a mask.

Thou has something stronger, a heart of gold.

Not only a heart of gold but one filled with gentle solicitous.

Her words fighting against my dreadful thoughts, words just words but more powerful than the monster trying to tear me down. Those words filled with mollifying reassurance.

Her reaching out to me, making sure I'm ok.

One small thing making me feel wanted for the first time. Making me feel hope something I haven't felt in years. I was no longer alone. I was fighting my battles but no longer alone, I had a champion by my side.

One that went out of her way and never gave up on me. A dedicated educator, no other can compare. Inspiring and motivating the hearts and minds of everyone around her.

A soul dazzling and gifted. In my eyes not another human like this.

A human so supportive.

So charming, a smile that is contagious.

So considerate, always a helping hand to give.

So hard working never taking a break until the job is done.

The words of who she is could go on forever, my hero an endless book of the help and courage she has given me.

Those remarkable words she said saved me.

Her reaching out, being so warm-hearted, saved my life.

The extraordinary hero, being so warm-hearted saved my life.

Her just being who she is saved my life.

I aspire to one day be like her, my hero Mrs. Brooks.

Savannah Kealey

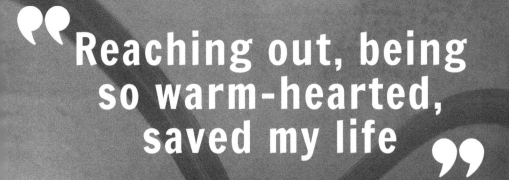

"Reaching out, being so warm-hearted, saved my life"

THINGS THAT HAVE PASSED ...

Your fingers, holding my top, fist curled to my chest,

Snuffling milk-drunk breath on my neck,

Midnight cuddles to chase away those dreams,

Little words mis-heard, mis-said,

The warm, solid weight of you asleep on my lap,

The fit of your head on my shoulder,

Your excitement at first times –

Swimming, bike-riding,

Swinging un-pushed, going for tea.

I'll keep it all safe for you,

Right here in these words.

By *Cate Haynes*

To ANYONE WHO NEEDS To SMILE –

Always smile at everyone is a rule I try to live by and a personality trait I have tried to instill into my three sons.

The saying "A smile is the most important thing you wear" rings very true to me. In a job where I interview people from all walks of life, from A-list celebrities to people going through harrowing times, smiling at them is the best way to connect. It not only breaks the ice but puts the person at ease.

Growing up as the daughter of a breast cancer surgeon, I was used to my father dealing with life and death on a daily basis. I would often ask him how he coped when treating his patients. It was his reply when I was probably in my late teens that stuck in my mind; he told me the importance of eye contact and a smile would often give them reassurance, faith and hope at a time when a cancer diagnosis obviously came as such a devastating blow.

So, I think, looking back, I then understood just how much a smile can work wonders. It makes you approachable, warm and kind. It can also help in stressful situations. From strangers on the tube and supermarket staff to colleagues, friends and of course loved ones, I always ensure

> I smile at everyone, even if it is not always reciprocated. If anything, it makes me feel like a better person.

In Dale Carnegie's famous book *How to Win Friends and Influence People* – which sold well over 30 million copies – the author felt smiling is so important that he devoted one entire chapter to the subject. And I cannot echo his words more; smiles radiate joy, excitement, confidence, health and vitality. Having lived through such uncertain times the past 18 months, that's what we all need right now!

By *Suzanne Baum*

SHOW ME

Show me a person who is afraid to die and I will show you a person that is yet to live!

By *A.F.J Drew*

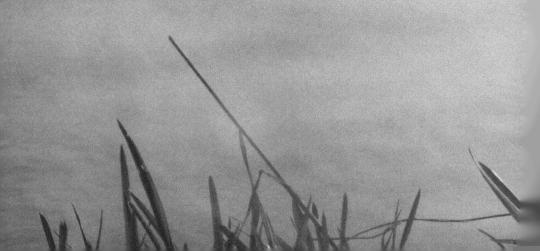

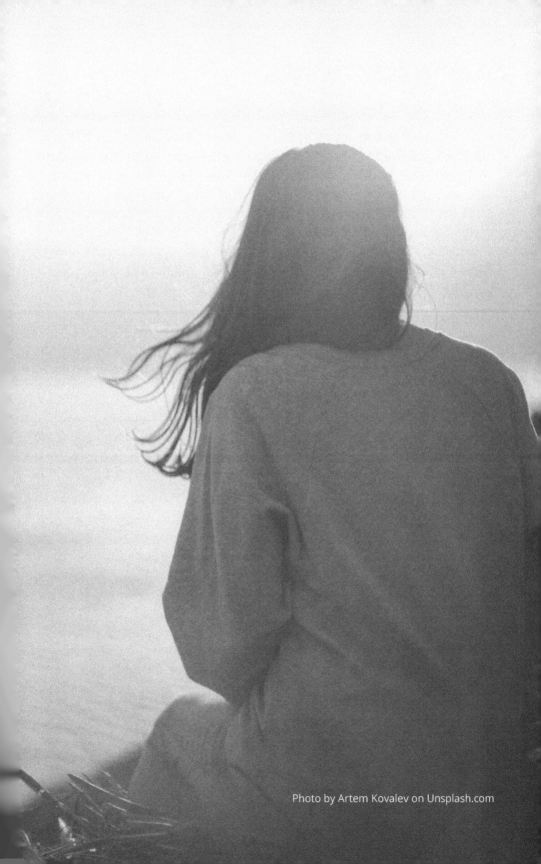

To MY (IN)SIGNIFICANT SELF –

Feeling pain is so subjective. When you feel stressed and emotional most often you start feeling butterflies in your stomach, which then leads to being sick, and then you start feeling the pain on your skin as if someone wounded you. When someone hurts you physically, what really hurts you is not the pain that comes from wounds. What hurts is the pain you feel in your heart because of what happened to you. You think less of yourself because you allowed that to happen to you, but you don't know how to make it stop. You think you haven't deserved it, but maybe you did. What do you know?

Well, it turns out you know everything! You are the only one that knows who you are and what you can become.

> You are the only one that can stop yourself from hurting. Because in the end, you choose what you are going to let get to you.

I was bullied, I was hurt, I was tortured, both physically and mentally. I felt useless, worthless, empty. I chose to feel like that simply by accepting that's all I am.

I failed to appreciate I was also loved, supported and had an amazing childhood. I had my best friend who would have always been there for me, but never told her how I felt. I've had both parents working very hard for us to have a future they knew they would never have. I thought they could never support me and understand me. I also failed to notice how madly in love they were because they were working so hard. I've had a very protective brother who would have done everything for me, but I didn't tell him because I was scared he would get hurt. I failed to see he would help me even though he was suffering more than me. Still, the 6 of us were living in two rooms and I wanted to help us all have a better life. The whole of my childhood I was working so hard to help everyone around me but would never ask anyone to help me.

By the time I grew up, my parents have made a life for me, so I never have to work so hard, making it possible for me to go to my studies. My

**You are the only
one that knows who
you are and what**
YOU CAN BECOME

brother survived the most difficult time in his life, after which he kept working so hard and found the strength to build his own company out of nothing but his creativity. My best friend has become the most beautiful person inside-out. She is my go-to person, who is always there for me, no matter what I need.

 It's funny how it is all about perception.

That's how I could choose to see my life, that is how it turned out. Instead, I felt there was always something missing from my life, and I let people keep hurting me. If only I had the strength to ask for help earlier.

I remember one time I was in real danger. In these situations, I think it is only natural to do what you are told and think about your wellbeing. But no, not me. It was me losing my head or my friend losing her dignity. She needed me and her dignity was everything I could think about. I was never the best person for myself, but I chose to be the best person to have around. I developed this need to be needed and feel useful no matter the cost. Connect that to me feeling useless in the past.

Everything that happened made me who I am today. I don't know if I would be a good person if people weren't so bad to me. I don't know if I would be so outspoken if I wasn't so quiet to begin with. Would I want to help others feel better if I never felt so bad myself? Would I know how to love if I didn't feel so unloved? Would I listen to others with such attention if I never started talking carefully myself? My guess is – I would not. I may be wrong. But how would I know to recognize that people are hurting if I wasn't hurt myself? How would I recognize they need to be helped if I didn't need help myself? How would I learn to be so enthusiastic about improvement, about someone's experience and satisfaction if I didn't feel how it is to be ignored about the same?

But I wish I didn't refuse to ask for help! I wish I realized earlier that the problem wasn't my body, my face, my height, my clothes, my attitude! The problem was that I wanted to seek my happiness in all the wrong places.

Past Ana would say: you are so useless you can't do anything right. You don't deserve to be happy. You shouldn't smile, because when you smile, you risk being twice as sad. You are a failure and can never be successful.

Today's Ana is saying: thank you past Ana. I am glad you felt so useless that you needed to make me want to make a difference. Thank you for teaching me I should smile even when I am not happy and thank you for teaching me to teach future Ana that it is even more ok to cry and accept you are not fine. Thank you for lasting long enough to allow me to become who I am today. I am successful at everything I do, even at making mistakes. Because I now learn from them.

Future Ana will say: thank you for teaching me it is ok to cry, accept you are not fine and ask for help. Thank you for being open, helpful and kind. Thank you for being a great role model for your son, your family, your friends and your colleagues. Thank you for making me so proud and for teaching others to lead your example and take pride in everything that happened to them. And last but not least – thank you for using the most difficult times you have had as the opportunity to keep learning and growing.

> Because in the end there is a silver lining in everyone's life, and everyone has the right to feel bad and good.

If you learn from everything good and bad that happened to you, you have had a successful life and if you have taught someone to do the same then you have made the difference.

Baby steps, small wins. REMEMBER – If you feel bad you can feel good, if you feel empty you can feel full. If you feel useless all you need to do is become useful. If you can feel sadness, then you deserve happiness as well. Take pride in everything you do and as long as you make mistakes – well done. Because that is how you learn and become successful. If mistakes are too deep and doing little things to make you happy doesn't work, ASK FOR HELP. That is a sign of true strength. And if the first person doesn't help that's fine because there is always a second, a third ... Be persistent until you have found your person and when you do make sure you appreciate them.

Ana Belic

TO WHOEVER NEEDS THIS –

If only I knew.

If only I knew the path before me,

Where it led, where to go and how to be.

If only I knew how to respond to change,

To make the right decisions and to do more than make do.

If only I knew working too hard was folly,

Worrying about things and forgetting to be more jolly.

If only I knew that life was so rich,

That living every moment was certainly not kitsch.

If only I knew that lives often are short,

Where every great moment should be enjoyed and caught.

If only I knew that that I was capable of more

That life was ever changing with opportunity for sure.

If only I knew that life was not just about work,

That working to live would prevent any hurt.

If only I knew that I could enrich other lives,

That through love and compassion I could help others to strive.

If only I knew there was no time to worry,

That happiness and fulfilment should never be hurried.

If only you knew what a life you will lead,

You'd know what fortune was in every great deed.

So, forget the worries and fears holding you back,

And know that your course is one on a great track.

To know your true greatness will take time and great strain,

That hardship comes with this, some difficulty and pain.

But be sure of one thing that is undoubtedly true,

A life of fulfilment and joy is waiting for you.

John Penquet

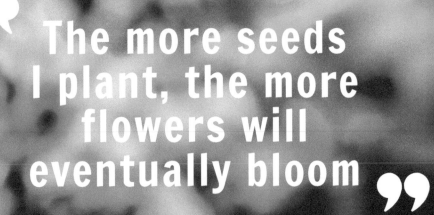

"The more seeds I plant, the more flowers will eventually bloom"

"DEAR MOM,

How are you?"

Jessica pauses, takes a sip of coffee, and looks at the sheet of paper in front of her. Then she shreds it to pieces, takes out a new one and writes:

"Hi Mom,

Sorry I haven't written in a while. But guess what? I have great news!

I got it, Mom! I got the job! They confirmed today.

I'm so happy. I can't fully believe it yet. But I'm proud of myself, I finally am! And I want you to be proud of me too.

Thank you, Mom. Thank you for everything you've given me and everything you've taught me.

You showed me that if I put in the effort, I'll inevitably see the results. And the more seeds I plant, the more flowers will eventually bloom.

There's been so many times when I got fed up with planting those seeds. Nothing would seem to take root. I thought there was something wrong with me. With me, Mom. Isn't that funny? Why hasn't it crossed my mind that something could've been wrong with the seeds or the soil? Or even the climate?

And then I remembered that summer at the beach, when I was 5 or so… You know, when we went to your friends' beach house? I was eating peaches and trying to plant the pits in the sand. And then I was checking on them every 10 minutes, terribly upset that they hadn't turned into trees yet."

Jessica smiles and shakes her head. Takes another sip of coffee and continues writing.

"And then you explained to me that it was the wrong place to plant them. We went to the garden, you let me dig holes and showed me how to plant them properly.

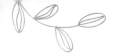

Later on, though, I also tried planting seashells in the sand - it somehow sounded logical to me. I'm not sure of the harvest I expected to see, but I have memories of drawing palm trees with shells instead of leaves in my sketchbook. You said I was a genius and wanted to frame it. But then we lost the sketchbook on the way back home.

What a funny kid I was.

What a lucky kid I was.

> **Your endless belief in me, in my talents, in my potential - that's what had always fueled me.**

That's why I never give up. That's why on the 1st of June I'm starting this new job.

What else...

Well, Matt and I—"

Jessica pauses. She looks at the letter, biting the tip of the pen. After finishing her cold coffee in one big gulp, she gets up, walks over to the sink, leaves the empty mug there, turns around and looks at the desk with the unfinished letter. Takes a few deep breaths, returns to the desk, picks up the pen.

"We visited Dr. Harrison last week. She still can't say anything for sure, she said she wanted to run some more tests. Said that we definitely shouldn't lose hope.

I don't want to lose hope, Mom. I don't want to lose anything or anyone anymore. I don't want to lose.

I just want a baby.

I want to be a mom. I don't know if I can be a mom like you, but I'll try my best. I'll give it my 1000%. I promise. I swear.

I want to plant peach pits and seashells with my kids. I want to read bedtime stories. Or make up some new amazing ones, like you did.

I want to teach them everything that I've learned from you. To share all I've got. To give all that I can. All that I am.

If only I'm given a chance."

A tear runs down Jessica's cheek and lands between the lines.

She takes a tissue out of the box, sticks its corner carefully into the teardrop, absorbing the salty liquid before it crawls on the letters. Then blows on the wet spot gently several times, so that it dries faster, wipes her face with another tissue, and continues writing.

"You know what, Mom, I'm going to have faith. I'll believe in it, stubbornly, just like you taught me.

I'll always remember how you said that if I want to use my stubbornness for something good, it should be believing in myself and my dreams, no matter what. It's no use believing in anything else, you said. And you were right.

You were right about so many things, Mom. I didn't always listen. I didn't always understand. I'm sorry, Mom. For all the times I've upset you. For all the times I was wrong but was too stubborn to admit it. For not listening. For not always being there. Please forgive me, Mom."

This time the tear lands exactly on the "M," turning it into a blot of ink.

Jessica takes another tissue, trying to save the situation, but it doesn't work. She gives up and decides to return to writing, before she makes an even bigger mess.

"I always start on a positive note and finish like this, don't I?

Well, consistency is king, as you always said. Haha…"

Jessica chuckles quietly.

"I need to go, Mom.

I just wanted to tell you that I love you so much. So, so much.

I also miss you so much it's hard to breathe, Mom.

I really need to go now.

I'll write soon.

Love you,

Your Jess"

Jessica puts the pen down, grabs another tissue, blows her nose loudly. Takes a long breath. Folds the letter carefully, takes an envelope, black with a gold trim, puts the letter inside, licks the flap and seals it.

She gets up, walks over to the fireplace and carefully places the envelope on top of the others that look just like this one, black with a gold trim, all neatly piled next to the urn with her mother's ashes.

Elena Carter

TO ANYONE WHO NEEDS TO TAKE A DEEP BREATH –

Breathing in, I am calm.

Breathing out, I detach from what I cannot control.

Breathing in, I am balanced.

Breathing out, I find clarity.

Breathing in, I am present.

Breathing out, I am whole.

Like the tides of the sea,

I move with the currents.

I do not grasp and fight,

But ripple and flow.

However life turns me,

I stay afloat.

Breathing here,

Breathing here...

Feeling it all.

Anonymous

HI DEBBIE,

I thought I would write you a quick note, as I did not want to disturb your journey.

I have followed your life as a foster carer for a while now and wanted to pass on the love and thanks for all you bring to fostering!

My parents have been foster carers for 11 years and I am now a social worker! I am actually travelling to Aberdeen to visit one of my lovely children who is in residential care!

How seeing the personal and professional perspectives of fostering, I have seen the utterly heart-breaking experiences of children. Often, we are left in a position wanting to do more but feeling contained by the social care system. BUT people like you are shouting from the roof tops about fostering, raising awareness and keeping children who are at risk at the front of everybody's minds!

Some days I am left feeling defeated, but people like you sincerely keep the hope and love alive!

So, thank you,

Georgia

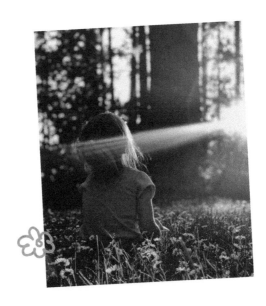

xdebbietowiex Kind gestures .... the power of a letter and the warmth of a human. Whilst I rushed around to board a plane to Scotland I sat back into my chair and sighed 😊. The last few years has had its fair share of emotions, along with the combination of lockdown, cancelled holidays, no schools, cancelled weddings and of course my babies moving onto their next chapters of life. I over the last month have reflected on life, cried, laughed and re charged my batteries which were running on reserve and some days in sorrow they were totally flat. As the flight took off I smiled ..... and then like a guardian angel a young lady dropped this note onto my lap, I had little chance to look up or catch a vision of a face, I just saw her a vision of a young lady heading towards the back of the plane. I carefully opened the letter, a simply kind gesture 🤍 but written with compassion and kindness. We must all be reminded occasionally that our ripples of love travels a million miles, thank you, you lovely lady you have made my day 🌻

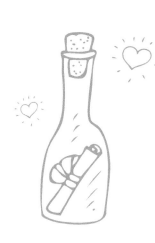

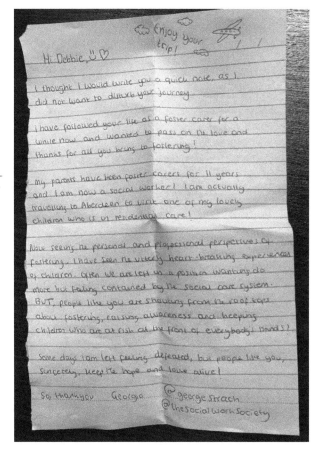

☁ Enjoy your trip! ☁ ✈

Hi Debbie, 😊 ♡

I thought I would write you a quick note, as I did not want to disturb your journey.

I have followed your life as a foster carer for a while now and wanted to pass on the love and thanks for all you bring to fostering!

My parents have been foster carers for 11 years and I am now a social worker! I am actually travelling to Aberdeen to visit one of my lovely children who is in residential care!

Now seeing the personal and professional perspectives of fostering, I have seen the utterly heart-breaking experiences of children. Often we are left in a position wanting do more but feeling contained by the social care system. BUT, people like you are shouting from the roof tops about fostering, raising awareness and keeping children who are at risk at the front of everybody's minds!!

Some days I am left feeling defeated, but people like you, sincerely, keep the hope and love alive!

So thankyou   Georgia   ☺ george strach
                                            @ The Social Work Society

DEAR PHILIP,

I hope, as do so many others, that somehow you find within you the strength to carry on. The courage you have shown since the day you were told you had cancer has been inspiring. If anyone can keep on defying the medical odds, you can.

But if this does defeat you this time, I don't want you to go without me saying what a wonderful person you are, and what an extraordinary friend you have been. Of all my friends, you are the one who touches virtually every point of my life – past, present, politics, work, leisure, sport and holidays, education, books, charity, and, more important than anything, family and friendship. I have been blessed to know you. So has Fiona. So have Rory, Calum and Grace. For so many of the happiest moments of our lives, you have been there, indeed often the cause of the happiness.

You've always been there in tough times too.

You remember the Alex Ferguson quote – "The true friend is the one who walks through the door when others are putting on their coats to leave." You have displayed that brand of friendship so often, so consistently, and with such a force as to keep me going at the lowest of moments.

When I got your moving, lovely message on Tuesday, and was convinced you wouldn't see out the night, I felt like a limb had been wrenched from me. You know my crazy theory that we only know if we have lived a good life as we approach its end – perhaps we only know the real value of a friend when we lose him. The loss for Gail, Georgia and Grace will be enormous. But so many others were touched by you and will share that loss.

My favorite quote of our time in government came not from me or you, or any of the rest of the New Labour team. It came from the Queen in the aftermath of the September 11 attacks ten years ago.

"Grief is the price we pay for love."

You are much loved. There will be much grief. But it is a price worth paying for the joy of having known you, worked with you, laughed with you, cried with you, latterly watched you face death squarely in the eye with the same humility, conviction and concern for others which you have shown in life.

I will always remember you not for the guts in facing cancer, brave though you have been, but for the extraordinary life force you have been in the healthy times. Your enthusiasm, your passion for politics, and belief in its power to do good, your love of Labour, your dedication to the cause and the team – they all have their place in the history that we all wrote together. I loved the defiant tone of your revised Unfinished Revolution, your clear message that whatever the critics say, we changed politics and Britain for the better. So often, so many of our people weaken. You never did. You never have. You never would. That is the product of real values, strength of character, and above all integrity of spirit.

In a world divided between givers and takers, you are the ultimate giver. In a world where prima donnas often prosper, you are the ultimate team player. Perhaps alone among the key New Labour people, you have managed to do an amazing job without making enemies. That too is a product of your extraordinary personality, your love of people and your determination always to try to build and heal. It has been humbling to see you, even in these last days and weeks, trying to heal some of the wounds that came with the pressures of power. We can all take lessons from that, and we all should.

Of course, I will miss the daily chats, the banter, the unsettled argument about whether QPR are a bigger club than Burnley. More, I'll miss your always being on hand to help me think something through, large or small. But what I will miss more than anything is the life force, the big voice. You have made our lives so much better. You are part of our lives, and you will be forever. Because in my life, Philip, you are a bigger force than the death that is about to take you.

Yours ever, AC

Alastair Campbell

Journalist, author, strategist, broadcaster

To ANYONE WHO COULD USE SOME ADVICE –

Here are ten things I've learnt about surviving as a foster carer.

1. Warmth and kindness always shines through. Smile. Because those who don't smile back need it the most.

2. Every single child that comes into your home will be scared. (wouldn't you be!) their fear will empty out in a million different ways.

3. No matter what journey they have travelled they will always love their family. Home is home.

4. Never go to bed on an argument...in your darkest moments tomorrow is another day.

5. Words are cheap actions are powerful. Show them you love them unconditionally. The simplest of gestures speak thousands of words.

6. There are always reasons for behaviors. It is about you finding them.

7. You will be many things ... a carer... a nurse... a friend ... a coach ... a teacher ... a therapist ... a night whisperer. Be prepared to wear many hats.

8. Educate yourself beyond every comfort zone you can imagine because to wear all these hats education is powerful.

9. Never judge. Never think you hold the answers. Sometimes there aren't any. It's called acceptance.

10. Love truly conquers all.

With love,

Debbie TOWIE (Instagram name @xdebbietowie)

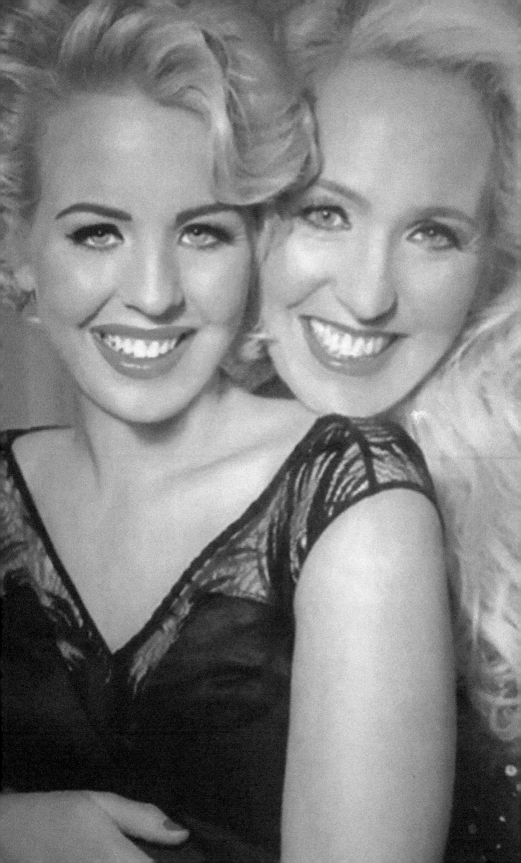

DEAR DARLING,

I loved you before you were born and now, you're growing up at a speed too fast for my comfort. My youth fading like the jumper washed too many times, as you become a brilliant young person. You're beautiful my darling, and your soul, mind and heart are equal in their beauty.

There are life lessons you'll learn; the positive, the detrimental and those you will teach others. There will be times in your life that feels like you are climbing a mountain wearing boxing gloves and tennis rackets as shoes. Times when everything seems out of your reach, too far to grasp and even see. Times that are painful, exasperating.

 Sometimes your inner strength will keep you going, soaring. Remember, the only failing is never trying.

Challenges will present in many forms. Friendships, relationships, choices. Sometimes, a split-second decision will have catastrophic consequences or be the best choice you ever made. Trust your gut instinct and realize none of us are immune from mistakes or bad times; instead they cultivate our growth. Information is empowering, assist people to build a box of tools to help themselves navigate through life. Don't keep giving advice that isn't listened too. Don't water dead plants.

Love equally. You'll be hurt by love; you'll hurt others in the path of love. Emotionally, physically, sexually, you should always feel equal in love. You'll may lose in love at some point. Lost love is still love. Never give up on love. True love is equal and feels like soul medicine. If you have a long-term relationship, make sure it's with someone who's your best friend and number one fan. Your true love is the first person you want to ring when something good or something bad happens. They're the person that makes you the best version of you. Accept nothing less. The person who gets to reciprocate your love will be the luckiest human alive! Never go to sleep on an argument. Never leave the house angry. Understand forgiveness. Don't always people please. Worry less and say no without guilt.

Show love and tell people they're loved. Hold loved ones tight. There will be a time when you can't hold them anymore. Where the void they leave feels like you're falling through space. Where a crack in your heart feels irreparable. The bad news is, it'll never fully repair. The good news is, is that the scar becomes part of who you are and your limp from their loss means you carry them with you, in your heart and mind. Keep birthday cards from people. Remember their smells, the touch of their skin, the way their home and presence make you feel. Take photos, capture memories in the snapshot of your heart.

Learn about your body. No one's ever happy with theirs, but your imperfections are perfectly you. Embrace your body, don't let other people judge it. Feed your body and soul with nutrition, respect, affirmations and sunshine. Don't abuse it with alcohol to the point of vomiting, it isn't big nor clever! Eat what you want, in moderation. Have a positive relationship with food. Cook, enjoy and indulge in food. Know your body. Know when things aren't right. Wear sunscreen to protect your pretty face and moisturize for eternal skin elasticity. Wear a sports bra when exercising and exercise until you feel the acid tang of breathlessness, it's an adrenaline like no other.

Laugh with friends, dance and joke. Enjoy your youthful innocence before routine and responsibility can become a pattern all too mundane. When you do have to adult, remember the inner child in you. The voice of fun and silliness. Never let that go quiet, it'll keep you and others sane in times of adversity. It will help you always see positives of our wonderful lives and world.

Be who you want to be and like what you like, as opposed to what you think you should from society's messages. Don't let stereotypes, expectations, stigma, media and other people dictate what you should do or who you should be.

Listen to your heart.

Our path can change directions as many times as we want. When you lose confidence, wear a mask until that confidence comes back. No one will know, except maybe those who know you the best and they'll always be your cheerleaders. Your mind won't always feel healthy. You are human. You'll have days that are struggles. Be kind to yourself.

Don't put pressure on yourself, the world will do enough of that to fill a reservoir, don't you contribute to the force. Get a job doing something you love.

Slow down, life isn't a race.

Intelligence isn't just I.Q. It is in the heart and emotional mind. It's the empathy you show others, your presence, your gratitude. Some of the most crucial life lessons include learning resilience, kindness and patience.

You will lose my darling. It is inevitable. You will lose friends, you'll fail tests, experience relationship break-ups and lose loved ones. I can't protect you from all of that, although I'll always be a blanket of reassurance and cuddles, no matter how old you are. Resilience will be your spine; it will hold you up and carry you through life. You're always stronger than you'll believe, and things always get better. I promise. Never be scared to ask for help. Sometimes reassurance can keep our lights shining.

The best things in life cost nothing. Money doesn't buy happiness; it allows you to have options that can make you happy. Choice, acceptance, equal love, safety and humor are the ingredients to happiness. Laugh. Sing songs that evoke memories of sheer joy. Make time to read books, they open a world of imagination and are your teachers. Travel. Visit new places and experience culture.

Be yourself my darling. Be kind, be proud, be funny and authentically you. Most importantly, love and respect yourself just like we do.

Helen Aitchison

xxx

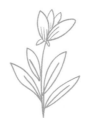

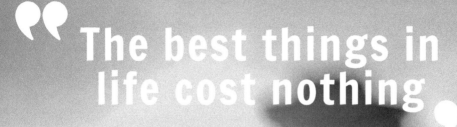

"The best things in
life cost nothing"

Dear, Fat Body

Feeling good about you isn't always easy. When I socialise with my slim family & friends, undress in front of my husband, go swimming or to a spa, I'm aware that people see you, before they see me.

You were thin once, before my mental health problems started. I was in control of you — I excercised regularly & ate sensibly. You looked good in clothes & people were attracted to you. You made me feel confident & respected.

Depression & anxiety mean't that I could no longer exercise or control you. You became bigger & bigger. Consequently, I feel that society perceives me as lazy & stupid. I wonder if some of the things that I do, I do to justify my place in the world. Do I do charitable things so that people will like me?

I have just turned 56, my mental illness is under control. I am lucky that I have a wonderful husband, family & friends & a job that I really enjoy. I have more control over you & I am more acceptant.

Although, my feelings for you are complex & sometimes contradictory, I feel like I am beginning to value you more.

I am starting to accept you for the way you are, & not the way that society tells us. I am happy about that.

Kind regards,

Me

248

DEAR FAT BODY,

Feeling good about you isn't always easy. When I socialise with my slim family and friends, undress in front of my husband, go swimming or to a spa, I'm aware that people see you before they see me.

You were thin once, before my mental health problems started. I was in control of you – I exercised regularly and ate sensibly. You looked good in clothes and people were attracted to you. You made me feel confident and respected.

Depression and anxiety meant that I could no longer exercise or control you. You became bigger and bigger. Consequently, I feel that society perceives me as lazy and stupid. I wonder if some of the things that I do, I do to justify my place in the world. Do I do charitable things so that people will like me?

I have just turned 56, and my mental illness is under control. I am lucky that I have a wonderful husband, family and friends and a job that I really enjoy. I have more control over you, and I am more acceptant.

Although my feelings for you are complex and sometimes contradictory, I feel like I am beginning to value you more.

I am starting to accept you for the way you are and not the way that society tells us. I am happy about that.

Kind regards,

Me.

DEAR AUNTY EILEEN,

Waking up to the mouthwatering smell of sizzling bacon drifting up from your kitchen was one of the highlights of my weekend when I was a young girl.

Lazing around in crumpled sheets on Saturday mornings, enjoying the slow lazy process of waking up, smiling as I realize that I don't have to get up early for school or church.

As I twist my back, stretch my neck and arms, I imagine you downstairs, in the kitchen, slicing the uncut bread into thick doorsteps with the pale-yellow handled knife. Buttering the bread with lashings of Lurpak butter, before putting the crispy bacon on top, then flattening the sandwich a little to make it easier for me to eat.

Tea is masting in the pot. I had one sugar in my tea, back then, so it tastes milky and sweet, and is just the right temperature to complement the bacon.

Friday nights at your house was also special. You allowed me to stay up late – sounds from The Torrens, horror films.

I know that you will be reading this letter, in heaven, with my mam and dad and hope you don't get into trouble.

Love,

Me

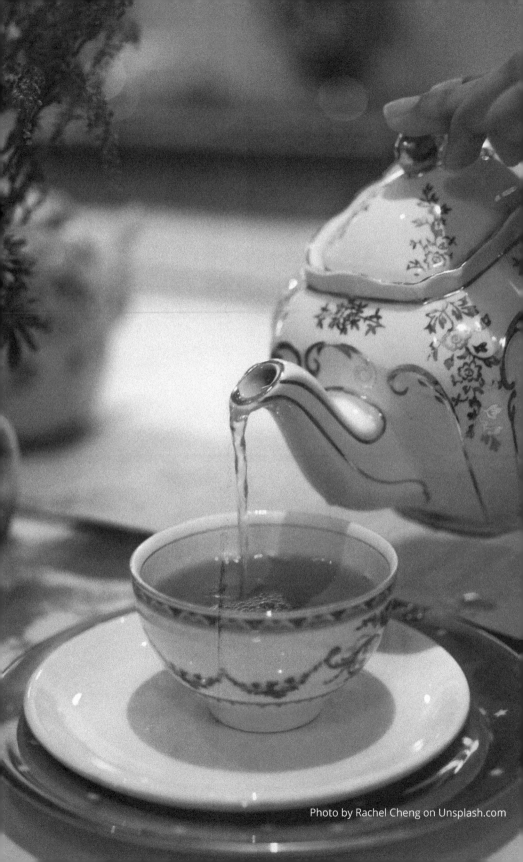

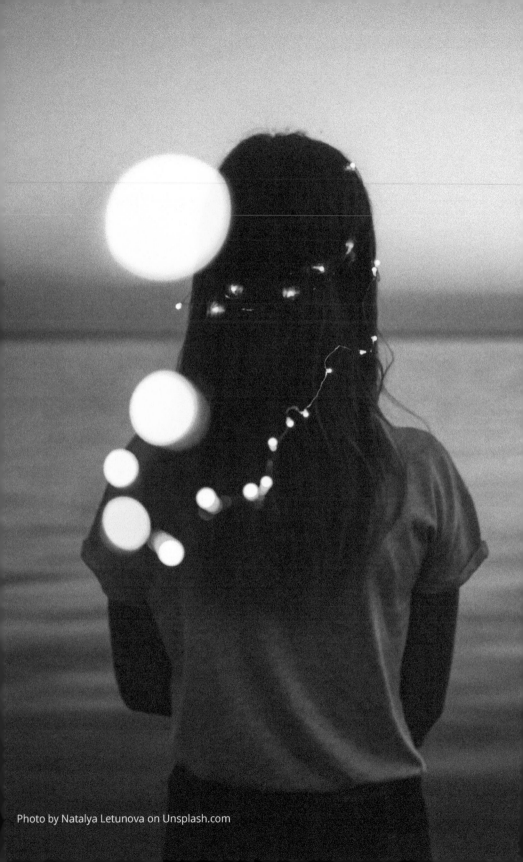

DEAR YOU,

When you were six, you wanted to be special. So, you wrote to the Tooth Fairy, asking them to make you magic. They never granted this wish.

When you were ten, you learned how to write in runes so you could put a spell above the window – something about dragons, to keep you safe. You hid it behind the curtain rail so no one would find out you were weird.

When you were a teenager, you swapped that childish protection for an armor of exam results, a cape of certificates, and finally, a professional helmet.

Now you are an adult, you wear those things still. Never mind: underneath, you're still weird. You write about hope and love and pain and sorrow, friendship and loss and wonder. You write about magic and weirdness.

> Because now you know: to be weird is its own kind of magic and the best armor of all.

Wishing you a lifetime of weirdness,

Cate Haynes

To ANYONE FEELING FEAR –

In my thirty years as a barrister there are plenty of times when I had fearful thoughts on the way to court. Because no matter how experienced you are, standing up in front of a judge is scary. I've had colleagues who used to throw up before going into court, one who fainted in the middle of submissions, and another who had a mental breakdown during a trial.

When I started out, I remember looking at senior barristers in their horsehair wigs and silk gowns and thinking that they must be different from me in some way. That their confidence and success were unattainable.

It took me a long time to realize that that was wrong.

The most important thing I learnt during my legal career was nothing to do with the law. It was that my colleagues, however eminent, were no different from me, and shared all the same fears. They just hid them better.

Although that realization helped, the fear never goes away. I've seen colleagues humiliated by judges. I've had my own submissions described as "hopeless," "misconceived" and "stupid nonsense." Sometimes you go to court knowing that the judge is going to hate your client and your submissions.

> But you go anyway. Because running away from your fears only makes them worse.

Tempting though it was, I never did step out in front of a car to avoid a difficult hearing. I came to appreciate that there would be good days and there would be bad days. Yes, there were times when I wished the floor could open up beneath me. And times when imposter syndrome struck – when I would look around court and wonder why twenty or more lawyers were spending all day listening to me cross-examining or making submissions.

You just have to get on with it and do the best job you can. If you've done that, then win or lose, you've dealt with your fear. You haven't conquered it. It hasn't gone away. It never will.

> *You need to learn to live with your fear, knowing that next time it will still be there.*

I've recently moved to a new profession – writing – where rejection is the norm. Yes, I've had a novel published, but I've suffered far more rejections than I can count. As has every writer. The fear of rejection can paralyze you. No one likes to be told that their work isn't good enough.

But I've realized that there is one thing that published writers have in common. Perseverance. The willingness to face their fears and go back again and again.

If you run from your fear, it gets bigger. It controls you. If you face your fear, it doesn't go away. But it becomes a little easier to deal with.

Guy Morpuss QC

Barrister and Author of *Five Minds*

RAINBOW HUES
by Ian Eagleton

There once was a boy who shone like the sun.

He sparkled and laughed with glee and with fun.

He was the color of a rainbow and marbled in love,

but soon life came crashing down from above.

Every day they would gather like wolves in a pack:

"You're weird, you're wrong, that's not how boys act."

"They don't dance and read, and they don't cry or sing!"

Then terror rained down as they lashed out at him.

He would beg and he'd cry and he'd sob and he'd plead.

"I'll go to a teacher – they'll know what I need!"

But Sir muttered and stuttered and spluttered and coughed:

"You're wrong, no it can't be! Go on… be off!"

Still, they continued to tease and to jeer.

What was it about him they so desperately feared?

So he thought and he pondered and concocted a plan,

on how he could be "A Typical Man."

He acted and tried, but life felt off key,

"I no longer feel happy – I no longer feel 'me'."

His colors had dimmed, now where had they gone?

Something had changed; they no longer shone.

Into the library he'd retreat and he'd hide,

a book in his hands, safely tucked by his side.

And from there he'd travel the world in a page,

searching for someone to show him the way.

Then one day it happened, he could take it no more.

They circled around him, but he stayed and he roared:

"You can kick me and hit me and mock me, then beat me,

but I cannot be stopped, no I won't be defeated.

For I'm strong and I'm brave and I'm kind and I'm wise,

I dance with the wind and I swim with the tides.

I am lit up by love, I am fierce and I'm free.

Your taunts and your sneers, they cannot harm me.

Many have suffered by your hands and your words.

They have cut and they've hurt, they have bruised and they've burned.

You have taken my colors, my voice you have stripped,

bound me and caged me, my wings you have clipped.

So listen to this and please listen well.

Come gather close, there's one last thing to tell:

If ever you touch me or hurt me again,"

he looked in their eyes, yes each one of them,

"then I'll fight back and rise up by just being me,

for I'm lit up by love, I am wild and I'm free."

Mouths open wide, they stopped and they stared,

at the Rainbow Boy shining, his soul finally bared.

Then they whimpered and shuffled, they turned and they ran.

"And if you come back, I am ready. I am!"

There are many ways to live, love and be

It's when we accept this, that we are finally free

So, that is the story of a boy I once knew,

And for all of the brave ones who fight to stay true.

MY DEAR MEL,

Are you sitting by the river again? It's a beautiful spot just there, I know. The view across the Mersey towards Liverpool is always spectacular. Sometimes the sun sparkles on the ripples, warms the golden stone and glances off the stark metal and glass. Sometimes scudding clouds reflect in the troubled depths as the city sulks and broods across the forbidding expanse of water. Sometimes the buildings only loom as mysterious silhouettes as swirling mists merge land into sky into tide. And yet there is always beauty to be found here. Is there any beauty in your thoughts today, Mel?

I know that often the water seems to echo your own feelings. Or is it simply that the mercurial river makes it possible for you to identify any element of your mood within? But Mel, I promise you that you won't find any solutions there. Is it a safe place for you today?

I see you as you perch on the edge of the wall, legs dangling free, mind entangled. You are solitary there, but you are not really alone.

You are surrounded by so much love.

And you do know it's there, but the frosted glass which so thickly divides you from the dimly-seen reality beyond prevents that love from reaching your heart. You know it, but you simply can't feel it. It's not a deliberate rejection. It's not a conscious reduction. You're numbed, dulled, deadened…

Are you safe, Mel? The relentless current is oblivious to your pain. It can't heal you. The nearby sea is not an escape route or a rescue plan. Its waves toss indifferent heads and spit spray unfeelingly into the thin, clear air. The stifling, suffocating brine wouldn't welcome you – wouldn't even notice your presence. But your absence would be keenly felt, Mel. Are you safe?

In time, you will learn to allow the flow of thoughts to follow the river's course away, away, away… The dangerous emotions will no more than lap gently at your feet before they disperse again. You will perch on the edge of the wall, legs dangling free, mind no longer entangled. The thick

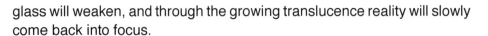

glass will weaken, and through the growing translucence reality will slowly come back into focus.

Many days you'll return here: alone; with friends; sharing; treasuring; pausing; lingering; brooding; exulting; watching the water reflect your emotions again.

> You'll see each aspect of the beauty before you, and you'll be aware of each facet of the beauty within you.

But Mel, while this is no refuge, while despair smothers all hope, while the impenetrable darkness of the present surrounds you and the future is a concept you can't even comprehend, come away. Come away from the river. Come away from its false pledges and fake assurances.

Look, Mel. Do you see? As you turn away from the glowering depths and you stumble faltering steps homeward, a mere hint of light silvers the edge of the menacing cloud above. The foreboding sky promises a hopeful rainbow. Not yet, but soon. Not yet, Mel, but soon. A hopeful rainbow, dear one. And then this will be a safe place for you once more.

Love,

Mel H.

To: EVERYONE THAT FEELS THAT YOU'RE JUST NOT GOOD AT ANYTHING IN PARTICULAR

From: Someone that feels like that more often than not and still gets sh*t done

"Mediocrity. The quality or state of being mediocre." That is how Merriam-Webster's dictionary explains how I felt most of my life, especially through that period in my life between 18 and 25 years of age, when you are supposed to find a calling, study to become "a professional" and get a job that streams out of that professionalism.

I never felt especially good at anything.

I hated sports, I was deeply introverted and loved sci-fi and fantasy novels. I never kissed a girl (I dreaded physical contact) until I was 18, and I had a couple (literally, two) friends. I didn't enjoy going to the movies with other people, and if I had my way, I would have spent more time inside my house than I actually did. I had no calling other than chatting online (and this was in the 90s, so it was nothing like your average chat experience these days), playing with my computer, and reading my books. My mother used to tell me that I had to study something, so I enrolled myself in a career I thought I would like but hated so I dropped out, coincidentally the same year my father died. That didn't help. I felt useless, and I felt neither friends nor family could help me so why would I even try to study or get a job?

I was sent away to travel, which of course for an introvert afraid of the world wasn't a great fix. Add that to the fact I was not good at traveling or getting to places or my own, or even talking to strangers and what you have is a panic attack waiting to happen far away from home. It did help though, and I realized that traveling had an unexpected meaning: no judgment could affect me. I was always a tourist so people wouldn't know if I was any good at anything or not. It was the perfect way of hiding what I considered back then to be the ultimate flaw, being mediocre.

Time passed, I eventually did enroll in a career I liked and even got a job out of it...only to realize (yes, you know it's coming) that I was not good at it and what was more important, for the first time in my life I decided

I didn't want to be any better at it. I could still use what I learned for something different, only I had to figure out what.

By then I had a few jobs as a tech support analyst. I took the graveyard shift, of course, it just made so much sense to me: late hours, the office was empty, and not a lot of people called tech support back then. I made good friends and learned a job (which my mother insisted I was a natural at because it was related to "that computer stuff you do"), but still, I felt like I was maybe average at it.

One day though I got a job in sales. I know, doesn't sound like something a guy that couldn't go get a haircut without blushing could do but it turns out it was a good idea. I still had severe problems building new relationships with people. It was stressful enough at first that I would come back home and sleep at least 10 hours every night, but after my first semester in the job something happened that I didn't even know how to process: I got an award.

It wasn't big or anything. Just your standard piece of carved glass that said, "Top Performer". Of course, that's a normal thing in sales, so normal no one keeps those pieces of glass but to me, it was life changing. How did it happen? I had no idea; I was only doing my job. Not humble-bragging, but reality: I had no clue how anyone could consider me a top performer at anything, especially as I felt literally everyone else did such a better job than I did at the same thing.

And then I got a second award, and a year later I got promoted. The basis for that promotion was consistent top performance, and I still didn't believe it. More importantly, I didn't feel it because let's be honest, we can all make ourselves believe something but making ourselves feel something is way harder. Have you ever tried falling out of love with someone by simply telling yourself to do so? Impossible.

That first promotion didn't change me, as much as the first award didn't either but what they did for me had set me in a different direction: I realized that feeling average doesn't really mean anything, at all. Other people would judge me the way they wanted, regardless of what I did. Some found me average, and I'm pretty sure some others just hated me but then some other people thought I was great, and they shared it with me. Those made a bigger difference but not because of the praise I got.

They proved something to me: sometimes how you feel matters the most, but sometimes it can limit you.

The problem with feeling mediocre is that it can convince you that you are just that, as if it was a bad thing or something despicable when, in reality, it is not. It is just a state, a way you feel. It doesn't even begin to describe or enable what you can achieve, and it has a secret power you might not be aware of: it is very persuading.

I don't know if you can stop feeling like that all because I sometimes still feel like that, especially when I am in the presence of people I deem way more intelligent than me, but I do know this thing: by all standards, I have failed at enough things in life to have learned a thing or two, and those things I learned allowed me to become who I am right now: a still very introverted public speaker, a sometimes-I-feel-like-I'm-not-that-good sales leader, a thought partner to C-level executives and a husband for almost 15 years as I write this letter. I can't say if those are great things or not to you, but I'm damn proud of them.

> If you feel anything like how I did I have just one piece of advice I will offer: be smarter than me and tell someone how you feel.

You might still feel the same way and it is ok, but you might also find out that what makes you unique is not how you feel, but how you overcome it.

Alejandro Cabral

"You might find out that what makes you unique is not how you feel, but how you overcome it"

LOVER OF THE MOON
By Alya Oliver

My sister once told me that

I find happiness in the saddest things:

Loving the scent of the dead autumn leaves,

Friends with the moon

Daughter of the wolves,

Craving the sight of rain falling through the sky.

Watching unnumbered twilights,

But not for their beauty,

But for the rising of the lady moon.

I told her I was different.

The sun would make me melt;

Loving the scent of the first snow,

Lover of the moon

Raised by wolves,

Frosting made me bloom.

I stopped chasing wingless birds,

But not for the nostalgia,

But for the rising of the true me.

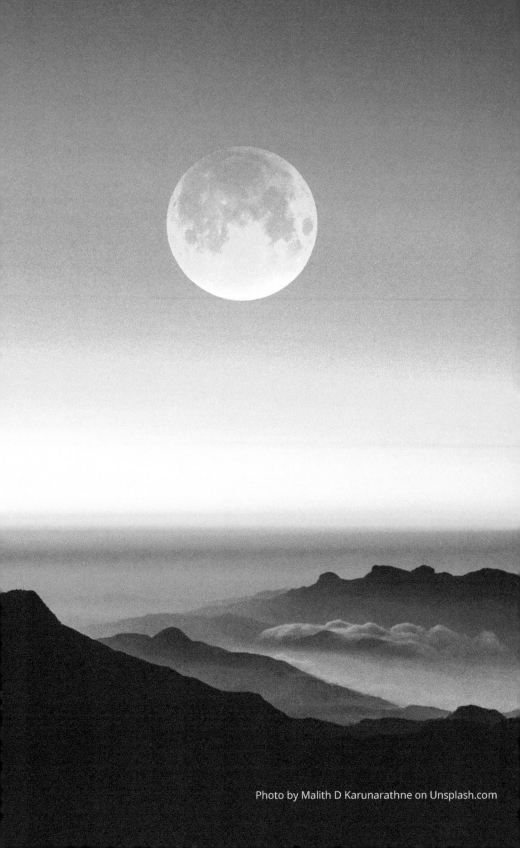

To ANYONE FEELING FEAR –

I have seen "the fear" in the eyes of many people!

Hold on, hold on, let me explain that before you start to get carried away with any sinister thoughts!

For many years, alongside my "normal" job, I have been fortunate enough to be an outdoor activities instructor, so things like climbing, abseiling, canoeing, mountain biking, mountain walking etc.

And during this time, I have seen many people being scared or nervous because they are faced with something outside of their comfort zone.

Whether it is a young person at the top of a 30 meter abseil, an experienced paddler at the top of a grade 4 rapid or indeed as I experienced a couple of years ago, a senior Vice President in the company I work for, just before he plunged himself into a freezing cold lake to do a capsize test in a kayak, they all had that moment where nerves or fear caught them.

This fear thing can be just a fleeting moment which is over in a flash, or it can be a more prolonged, drawn out, debilitating thing which is tremendously difficult to overcome and, in some cases, of course it stops us completely.

These feelings are not just caused by extreme activities, fear can grip us in many situations, starting a new venture, doing a task at work which is different to your normal tasks, pitching a new idea to someone or even starting that first conversation with someone new, fear can grip us anywhere.

> And it doesn't matter who you are, how old you are, what position you hold at work or what your background is, fear can creep up on you at any time.

Now, I don't have a magic potion to stop people having "the fear", but what I can say is unless you try different things, the fear becomes stronger and therefore more difficult to control.

I have seen the experienced paddler navigate the technical grade 4 rapid and then go and do it again and again to refine his lines and increase his speed.

I witnessed the 14-year-old girl finally descend the abseil after hesitating for 10 minutes before she stepped over the edge. She screamed all the way down, but the screams of fear turned into screams of joy halfway down when her worst fears were not realized, and she wasn't going to die!

And you should have seen the massive grin on the face of the senior Vice President when his head emerged from the cold water of the lake following his capsize test.

But it isn't just about the initial buzz of doing the thing which gave you the fear, no it's much more than that, overcoming fear prepares you, it trains your mind to be able to deal with fearful situations in the future and the more you do it the more you can control the fear rather than it controlling you.

> Believe me, no matter how experienced you are, whether it be at extreme activities, a senior leader in business or indeed at life in general, the fear is always there and learning how to control it and use it to your advantage is a key ability.

I am sure that there are many books or Internet articles about how to overcome fear, so if you are really interested in this area, there will be many resources you can get, but for me the quickest and easiest way to start controlling the fear is to just go ahead and take the plunge!

Good luck!

Ian Barnes

DEAREST YOU,

It hits you, the bite of the cold crisp air. You inhale a deep breath, and it starts to recharge your senses. As you exhale the mist of breath creates a cloud, a moving creation of transparent white foamy speckles that takes on a living form of its own. Full of CO_2 it's how your body naturally empties what it doesn't need. I shut the door behind me.

I always look back and then around when I leave home for my walk. Somehow, I always feel so lucky to be able to do that. Meant to be such a simple act, not everyone does walk or can. I'm always grateful for what I have until you think things will no longer be or you lose them, I wish no one the mutter of "if only I had" we all know recent events around the world brings that into sharp focus.

Crunch, crunch. The squelching noise of the pebbles beneath my feet make such a funny loud sound. It alerts people nearby, like a foghorn announcement that you are there. Sometimes I don't want people to know my presence, my wish to walk by without being noticed, to silently glide past as I see a couple deep in conversation. Instead, I disturb them, the look on their faces startled, we glance at each other. A silent comment exchanged, no words spoken, a simple nod of the head and smile from me seals the respect. Strangers connecting, feelings exchanged, a presence understood without a murmur, in slow motion and not a pretend.

The tall grass hides the path ahead. Crunch again… but this time I know it's a snail. I've accidentally stood on it. I say a prayer. I don't ever mean to do that but can't help what I can't see in the undergrowth. So beautiful it stands tall, the green and light strands of grass move like a symphony conductor's wand.

"Hello, you," a butterfly comes to visit, to check out what's happening and then delicately flitters away. A beautiful creature, elegant and light, small, yet was born from a magnificent creation out of a caterpillar – what a delight. A beautiful wonder that simply happens. Mother Nature doing her thing with hidden secrets and treasures, only she knows and turns the key to her creations.

> The ripples will travel far and wide and you will be glad as your very own adventures mark their place

The path ahead seems long, I've done this walk so many times, I should know by now it's shorter than it first appears. The unknown seems scary, even on a trodden path before me. It's amazing how we think when we can't see something ahead, why always it fills us with dread?

My heart was racing and the colour in my cheeks was so red. I'm excited and out of breath, funny how this is the dance that eliminates all that unnecessary dread. What an achievement, with just a simple step, one foot in front of the other, repeat that until you reach an end or wait for your trusted bleep to sound, from your digital friend.

Shoes off and back indoors. Beads form that glistens my neck. A big in-breath and then exhale, I stand in the hallway and it's like you've achieved something surreal. Was that an "out of body experience?" I ask myself. Nope, just my walk that helps me to remember the world I live in and to be grateful for what you have, big or small.

> Amazing adventures can be had from ordinary things, but if only you looked closer you would see and maybe even imagine, how extraordinary they are.

Look in the mirror, smile and say thank you for what you see. No need to speak out loud if you don't feel that's quite in line with how you feel. But what you can do is take a moment to look, really look at what you see. Each crease and facial feature tell a unique story of its own. The tales you could share, rich or poor will be worth it, as they are yours and my beautiful friends, who read this letter, you are all worthy in this small world. Please don't wait for others to tell you that, that's the energy you need and anything negative doesn't matter.

Do it now, akin to throwing a pebble in your lake and watch the adventures you will create. The ripples will travel far and wide and you will be glad as your very own adventures mark their place.

With love,

Hina Sharma

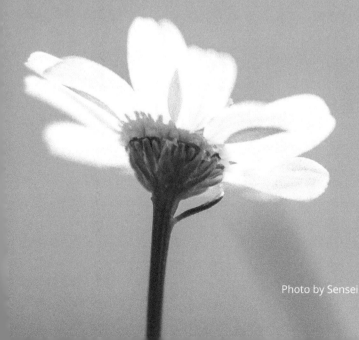

Look in the mirror, smile and say thank you for what you see

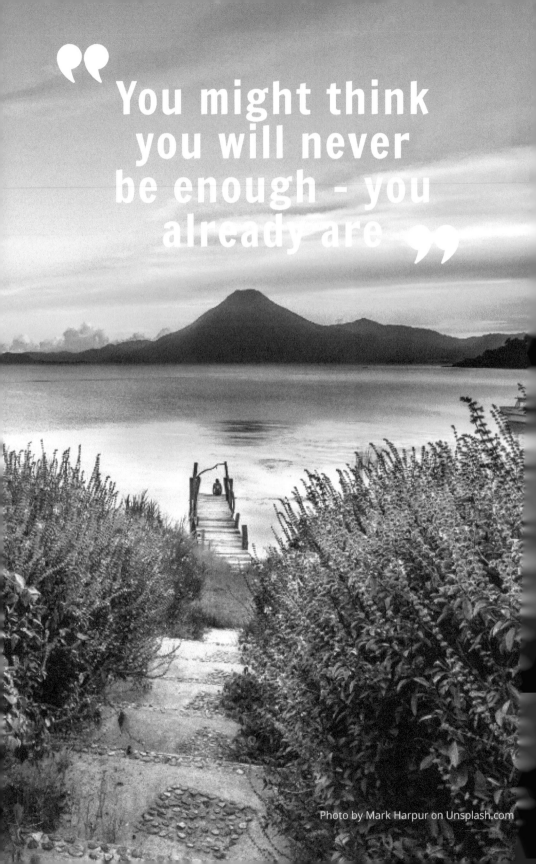

"You might think you will never be enough - you already are "

DEAR YOU,

You might think you can't do it - you can.
Think about all the times you did it before.

You might think you aren't good enough – you are.
You are a light for some people and you don't even realize it.

You might think others are better than you – they aren't.
They are thinking the same as you most likely.

You might not think you can get through the day – you can.
You've made it through every bad day up to now, so keep going.

You might think things won't get better – they will.
Maybe not today or tomorrow but they will at some point.

You might think they don't feel like you do – they do.
They are just hiding it well as you try to do.

You might think you will never be enough – you already are.

Be you and be kind to you.
You might surprise yourself!

Kyrstie Stubbs

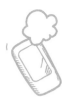

USEFUL NUMBERS

Here is a list of organizations and helplines to use if you find yourself in need of support. These are a small sample taken from The Prince's Trust website, which has a wealth of resources.

Check them out at **www.princes-trust.org.uk**

International Youth Foundation

The International Youth Foundation mobilizes a global community of businesses, governments, and civil society organisations – who are each committed to developing the power and promise of young people.

https://iyfglobal.org/

Livity

Livity gives ambitious young people access to creative opportunities through workshops, co-working space, exhibitions and more.
020 7326 5979

https://livity.co.uk/

The Mix

The Mix is the UK's leading support service for young people. They can help you take on any challenge you're facing - from mental health to money, from homelessness to finding a job, from break-ups to drugs. Talk to them via their free confidential helpline. 0808 808 4994

https://www.themix.org.uk/

The Samaritans

The Samaritans provide round-the-clock support for those in need, via their free helpline. 116 123

https://www.samaritans.org/

Youth Business International

Youth Business International provides thousands of young entrepreneurs with an integrated package of support to help them start and grow sustainable businesses. 020 3326 2060

https://www.youthbusiness.org/

Disability Rights UK

Disability Rights UK is the leading charity of its kind in the UK, run by and for people with experience of disability or health conditions.
020 7250 8181

https://www.disabilityrightsuk.org/

Mental Health Foundation

Mental Health Foundation is the biggest, most comprehensive website on mental health in the UK.

https://www.mentalhealth.org.uk/

Mermaids

Mermaids provides support for families, teens and children with gender identity issues.

National Trans Youth Network

https://mermaidsuk.org.uk/

Stonewall

Stonewall empowers individuals in the UK and abroad by providing them with support and advice to help tackle discrimination and hate crimes. As well as campaigining for greater equality, it has a range of research and resources to support you. 020 7593 1850

https://www.stonewall.org.uk/

Cruse Bereavement Care

Cruse Bereavement Care is a national charity offering counselling, support, help and advice to the bereaved. 0808 808 1677

https://www.cruse.org.uk/

Anti-Bullying Alliance

Anti-Bullying Alliance is a coalition of organisations and individuals that are united against bullying.

https://anti-bullyingalliance.org.uk/

Men's Advice Line

Men's Advice Line provides support for men experiencing domestic violence. 0808 801 0327

https://mensadviceline.org.uk/

National Domestic Violence Helpline

National Domestic Violence Helpline provides a free 24-hour emergency helpline. 0808 200 0247

https://www.nationaldahelpline.org.uk/

Mind

Mind provide advice and support to empower anyone experiencing a mental health issue. They campaign to improve services, raise awareness and promote understanding. 0300 123 3393

https://www.mind.org.uk/

Smokefree

Smokefree is an information service for those who are serious about quitting smoking, providing kits to remain smoke free as well as support via text and email. 0800 022 4332

https://www.nhs.uk/better-health/quit-smoking/

The Prince's Trust also work with local partners around the world to deliver education, employment and enterprise programmes that empower young people to learn, earn and thrive. These programmes are present in 13 countries within the Commonwealth and beyond across Asia, Africa, the Caribbean, the Middle East and Europe.

More details can be found at **https://princestrustinternational.org/**

ACKNOWLEDGEMENTS

Two simple words are all it takes.

It's something that we say every day for various reasons and the impact that it has on somebody else's day is different for each person. It's such a simple thing with so much behind it. For the person saying it, it shows gratitude and appreciation for something done. An acknowledgement that you've taken the time to do something to help somebody else. For the person receiving it, it's knowing that your actions have made a difference, no matter how small, and that you have had a positive impact on that person.

So, from all of us at Team Inspire, we would like to say a very heartfelt thank you and to give a special shout out to the following people who behind the scenes helped us and inspired us to drive forward with this project and campaign.

Thank you to our business mentor Valentin Bula, your creativity and entrepreneurial mindset was valued more than we can say.

To our executive sponsor at Pitney Bowes, Ryan Higginson who made this unique opportunity for Team Inspire possible. Gary Abbott for your help and guidance throughout. To Angela Holland and The Prince's Trust team thank you.

Team Inspire also wish to say thank you to Lawrence Maynard, Paul Lewis, Paul Crang, Claire Fincham, Greta Wilson, Kathleen Ryan Mufson, Polly Morrow, Deborah Kinsella, Christopher Johnson, Samson Okpanachi who supported us in their own special way with their expertise, resources and time, to other Pitney Bowes colleagues too many to name, you know who you are and fellow team member Rory Hannigan – thank you.

To our family and friends who put up with us throughout the many seasons we went through to create The Power of Letters, book.

We are sincerely grateful to our editor Jesse Lynn Smart for her judgement and editing services, and Lynda Mangoro, our brilliant book designer, for bringing everything to life and for her care to design with each story. To the magical Nicola Humber for your inspiration and introducing Jesse and Lynda to us and to all the photographers from Unsplash.com (listed throughout this book) who have donated their work for free.

To our contributors and followers, who took the time to share their stories and letters. Thank you for opening your hearts so that others can share in your experiences and sharing with your networks and followers.

To everyone who donated money to The Prince's Trust. You will be helping young adults facing challenges step into the world and make their mark.

Thank you to all of you for giving us your stories, your ideas, your time and your inspirational words of encouragement. It is your inspiration that will carry these encouragements forward.

With love,

Team Inspire

ABOUT TEAM INSPIRE

We came together working as an independent group of people to raise money solely for The Prince's Trust as part of the Million Makers campaign. We volunteered our personal time to create something that we believe can help support the young and old whenever needed.

This is our small way to connect people around the world, our hope and belief is that our collection of letters and poems will support those facing challenges to step into the world and help them make their mark, inspire many to believe in the power of a positive mindset, to learn from real life experiences, and show what can be possible.

In case readers wanted a musical inspiration, we thought we would share one of our favourite "lift me up" song titles. Ones that you couldn't help tapping your toes or dancing to, especially when no one was looking to share joy.

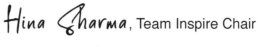

Hina Sharma, Team Inspire Chair

Led the team throughout the fund-raising challenge and campaign.

"Shine" by Take That

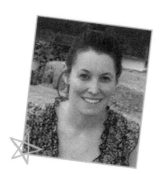

Gillian Willows, Logistics lead, social media outreach on Twitter and team support.

"9-5" by Dolly Parton

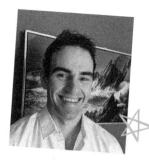

Mirza Mehmedovic, Business plan, finance lead and team support.

"Lovely Day" by Bill Withers

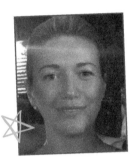

Laura Bunyan, Social media lead and team support.

"Truly Madly Deeply" by Savage Garden

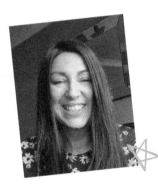

Vanessa Parker, Communications lead and team support.

"I'm Your Man" by Wham

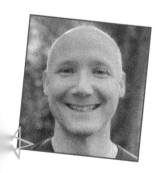

Darryl Thole, Creative Writer and team support.

"Hold my hand" by Hootie & the Blowfish

WWW.THEPOWEROFLETTERS.COM

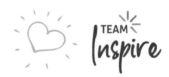

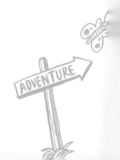

Lightning Source UK Ltd.
Milton Keynes UK
UKHW050958040722
R3096700001B/R30967PG405252UKX00001B/1